Biophoton Quantum Nutrition

A Breakthrough in Nutritional Science

James Z Liu, MD PhD

Biophoton Quantum Nutrition:
A Breakthrough in Nutritional Science

ISBN Paperback: 979-8-89576-152-6

Published by:

AUTHORS on MISSION

Preface

Biophoton Quantum Nutrition: A Breakthrough in Nutritional Science

For centuries, human beings have sought health, vitality, and longevity through food. Modern nutrition has made invaluable advances, discovering vitamins, minerals, cataloging macronutrients, and designing dietary frameworks to prevent deficiency and disease. Yet despite this progress, the global rise of chronic illness, fatigue, and age-related decline continues. Even among the most disciplined patients and high-performing individuals, I have observed persistent struggles with energy loss and cellular degeneration.

These observations led to a critical realization: an essential dimension may be missing from our current understanding of nourishment.

This book begins with two questions: *What if food is more than chemistry? What if we have overlooked the light?*

Years of research in quantum biology, biofield science, and photonic medicine revealed a new paradigm: light is not only a source of energy, but also a carrier of biological intelligence. Our cells both emit and absorb biophotons—ultraweak photons that regulate DNA activity, mitochondrial function, and intercellular communication. These subtle light-based interactions are not peripheral; they are foundational to life itself.

From this discovery emerges the field of Biophoton Quantum Nutrition: an integrative approach that views nourishment not merely as molecules, but as light, frequency, and information. In these chapters, you will explore how biophoton-rich foods restore coherence in the body, how structured water and electromagnetic harmony influence vitality, and how light-based technologies can revitalize metabolism, support detoxification, and even slow or reverse biological aging.

This book is both scientific and practical. It provides theory grounded in research, while also offering tools for everyday living:

- Meal planning strategies that emphasize high-photon foods.
- Environmental practices to align your rhythms with natural light cycles.
- Quantum-enhancing devices that amplify cellular coherence and resilience.

Whether you are a clinician, a wellness practitioner, or someone seeking personal transformation, this book was written for you.

We are living in an era marked by chronic stress, environmental toxicity, and increasing disconnection from nature. The call to nourish ourselves more deeply has never been greater. *Quantum nutrition* invites you to go beyond calories and molecules, and to embrace a model of health rooted in light, coherence, and consciousness.

May these pages remind you of a truth that has always been within reach: you are not only what you eat; you are what you radiate.

James Z. Liu, MD, PhD
Author and Biophoton Therapy Researcher

Dedication

To Professor John A. Milner, PhD—
Former Professor at Pennsylvania State University,
Forever Mentor, Tireless Advocate for Scientific Integrity,
and a Beacon of Wisdom in the Field of Nutrition and Health.

Your unwavering guidance, intellectual rigor, and deep humanity
shaped not only my scholarship but the very path of my life.
This work is a tribute to your legacy,
and to the enduring mentorship that continues to inspire every page.

Milestones in Nutritional Sciences

Introduction

The science of nutrition has evolved through centuries of observation, experimentation, and technological innovation. From early dietary theories rooted in balance and humoral medicine to the cutting-edge exploration of biophotons and quantum biology, the discipline has continuously expanded its scope. Each milestone reflects humanity's growing understanding of food not only as sustenance but as a carrier of energy, information, and healing potential.

1. Ancient Foundations: Food as Medicine

- Ayurveda and Traditional Chinese Medicine (2000 BCE–500 BCE): Early traditions emphasized food's energetic qualities, linking diet to balance, health, and longevity.
- Hippocrates (460–370 BCE): Famously stated, "Let food be thy medicine." This framed diet as central to health management.

2. The Age of Discovery and Deficiency Diseases (1500s–1800s)

- Scurvy and Vitamin C (18th Century): Sailors' recovery through citrus fruits revealed the role of specific foods in preventing disease.
- Pellagra, Beriberi, and Rickets (19th Century): Deficiency diseases highlighted the importance of micronutrients.

3. Birth of Modern Nutrition Science (1900–1950)

- Discovery of Vitamins: The identification of vitamins A, B-complex, C, D, E, and K established the foundation of micronutrient science.

- Calorie Theory and Energy Balance: Quantification of energy intake and expenditure redefines dietary planning.
- Protein and Essential Amino Acids: Grounded the role of macronutrients in growth and repair.

4. Nutrition and Public Health (1950–1990)

- Dietary Guidelines: Governments developed food pyramids and recommended daily allowances.
- Chronic Disease Connection: Research linked diet with heart disease, diabetes, and obesity.
- Rise of Industrialized Food: Advances in preservation, fortification, and mass production shaped modern eating patterns.

5. Nutrigenomics and Systems Nutrition (1990–Present)

- Nutrigenomics: Exploration of how diet interacts with genes to affect health outcomes.
- Microbiome Research: Recognition of gut bacteria as critical players in metabolism, immunity, and mental health.
- Functional Foods and Supplements: Growing focus on bioactive compounds beyond essential nutrients.

6. The Quantum Frontier (21st Century and Beyond)

- Biophoton Research: Evidence that cells emit ultra-weak light, linking food freshness and vitality with photonic emissions [Popp, 1992; Van Wijk, 2005].
- Structured Water and Quantum Biology: Food is seen not only as chemical fuel but as structured information that modulates coherence in living systems [Pollack, 2013].
- Biophoton Quantum Nutrition: A new paradigm integrating light, frequency, and consciousness into dietary science, positioning coherence as the ultimate measure of nutritional quality.

Summary

Nutritional science has traveled from ancient wisdom through modern biochemistry to the frontier of quantum biology. Each milestone reflects a shift from focusing solely on material molecules to acknowledging energy, frequency, and light as integral dimensions of nourishment. The future of nutrition lies in merging classical frameworks with quantum perspectives to cultivate health, longevity, and coherence.

Foreword

For more than a century, modern biology has been guided by a reductionist lens, dividing the body into its constituent molecules, calories, and quantifiable parts. Nutrition evolved in parallel, emphasizing proteins, fats, carbohydrates, and vitamins as the essential building blocks of health. This paradigm has generated remarkable advances, but today it is reaching its limits.

At the edges of science, a new understanding is taking shape. It is becoming clear that light, frequency, coherence, and quantum fields are not peripheral to life; they are fundamental. The human body is not only a biochemical system but also a bioenergetic one. Our cells communicate not only through chemical messengers but also through faint pulses of light known as biophotons. Structured water, vibrational resonance, and electromagnetic harmony are emerging as equally vital to human vitality as any known nutrient.

This book, *Biophoton Quantum Nutrition: Nourishing the Body with Light, Frequency, and Consciousness,* arrives at a pivotal moment. It challenges us to expand our definition of nourishment and introduces a bold but evidence-based proposition: that biophotons—ultra-weak light particles emitted by living cells—function as quantum nutrients. This insight, far from being an abstract theory, resonates with ancient traditions that recognized food as a carrier of life force, *qi,* or *prana.*

The author skillfully bridges quantum biology, nutritional science, and integrative health into a unified framework. Each chapter synthesizes rigorous research with timeless wisdom and offers practical applications that are both empowering and deeply respectful of the body's innate intelligence. The protocols are not just techniques; they are invitations to reconnect with our own light.

This work is more than a scientific contribution; it is a reawakening of an intuitive truth long forgotten that we are beings of light, and light is our food.

As a researcher and physician who has devoted decades to studying the intersections of energy, biology, and consciousness, I believe this book marks the dawn of a new era in medicine and nutrition. It shows us that food is not merely fuel; it is also frequency, coherence, and information.

Let this book guide you toward deeper vitality, radiant longevity, and an enduring sense of connection with life itself.

Xinying Lin, Professor, Nutritional Sciences

Contents

Preface 3
Dedication 5
Acknowledgements 6
Milestones in Nutritional Sciences 7
Foreword 10

Part I: Biophoton Quantum Nutrition— A New Era 17
Chapter 1: What Is Biophoton Quantum Nutrition? 20
Chapter 2: Quantum Nutrients 28
Chapter 3: The Biophysics of Life 37
Chapter 4: Biophotons—Light Within Living Cells 45
Chapter 5: The Biofield and Nutritional Resonance 52
Chapter 6: Academic Teaching—Biophoton Quantum Nutrition ... 60
Chapter 7: Scientific Research in Biophoton Quantum Nutrition ... 66
Chapter 8: Biophotons and Consciousness 74
Chapter 9: Biophotons and Frequencies in Nourishment 84

Part II: The Quantum Nature of Nutrients 91
Chapter 10: Food as Information 93
Chapter 11: The Photon Profile of Living Foods 100
Chapter 12: Water, Structure, and Light 107
Chapter 13: Sunlight as a Master Nutrient 116
Chapter 14: How to Combine Biophoton Exposure 123

Chapter 15: How to Measure Progress and Biological Age Reversal 131
Chapter 16: How Biophotonic Medicine May Reshape Aging, Longevity Clinics, AI-Assisted Diagnostics, and Global Wellness Systems 139
Chapter 17: Deglycation and Detox with Quantum Inputs 147

Part III: Practical Quantum Nutrition 155
Chapter 18: Building a Biophoton-Rich Diet 157
Chapter 19: Quantum Meal Planning 163
Chapter 20: Integrating Biophoton Devices in Daily Life 169
Chapter 21: Quantum Nutrition for Pets 176
Chapter 22: Quantum Nutrition for Plants 181
Chapter 23: Quantum Nutrition in Medicine and Longevity 187
Chapter 24: AI, Frequency Mapping, and Personalized Nutrition . 196
Chapter 25: Rewriting the Human Health Paradigm 203
Chapter 26: Living as a Quantum Being 211
Chapter 27: Mitochondrial Deficiency Is a Kind of Biophoton Deficiency 218
Chapter 28: Biophoton Deficiency and Lack of Coherence Are the Causes of the Most Common Disorders 227
Part IV: Commercial Usages of Biophoton Quantum Nutrition 235
Chapter 29: Biophotons Increase Students' Learning and Testing Performances 237
Chapter 30: Biophoton Energy Reduces Fatigue and Improves Working Performance 243
Chapter 31: Biophotons Energize Athletes to Improve Competitiveness 249

Chapter 32: Biophoton Energy Enhances Horse Racing Performance...256
Chapter 33: Biophoton Energy Increases Food Quality...262
Chapter 34: Biophotons Increase the Yield of High-Value Agricultural Crops...269
Chapter 35: Biophotons Increase Fermentation for the Wine Industry...277
Chapter 36: Biophotons Increase Fermentation for the Pharmaceutical Industry...284
Chapter 37: You Are Light—Feed the Light...292

Appendices...298
Food Biophoton Emission Index (Selected Examples)...302
Suggested Reading and Resources...305
About the Author...308

PART I

Biophoton Quantum Nutrition—A New Era

This section introduces the foundational principles of Biophoton Quantum Nutrition, a new paradigm that redefines food and health through the lens of light, frequency, and coherence.

Chapter 1 reframes nutrition beyond calories and molecules, exploring how food also serves as a carrier of biophotons and vibrational information.

Chapter 2 introduces quantum nutrients, subtle energetic and informational inputs that nourish the body at a cellular and field level through digestion, absorption, metabolism, biological function, and excretion.

Chapter 3 lays out the biophysics of life, showing how biological systems operate as quantum fields regulated by coherence, resonance, and electromagnetic order.

Chapter 4 explores biophotons, the ultra-weak light emitted by living cells, as regulators of DNA activity, mitochondrial efficiency, and cellular communication.

Chapter 5 expands this view to the biofield, the body's organizing energy field, and explains how nutritional resonance supports coherence across organs, tissues, and consciousness.

Chapter 6 examines how academic teaching in nutrition must evolve, integrating biophoton science into education to prepare future practitioners and students for this new era.

Chapter 7 explores the importance of rigorous scientific research in advancing the field of *biophoton nutrition.* It reviews key experimental findings, introduces emerging methodologies, and highlights new interdisciplinary directions that integrate biology, physics, and nutrition science.

Chapter 8 examines the relationship between *biophotons and consciousness,* emphasizing how cutting-edge research connects light-based cellular communication with neural coherence, cognition, and higher states of awareness.

Chapter 9 uncovers the role of *biophotons and frequencies in quantum healing,* illustrating how light and vibrational information work together to restore coherence, promote regeneration, and support holistic health at the most fundamental level.

Taken together, these chapters provide a comprehensive framework for understanding how nutrition in the 21st century must evolve from a reductionist focus on molecules to a quantum-informed model that honors the energetic intelligence of life. Part I establishes the intellectual and scientific foundation for the practical applications explored in later sections of the book.

Core Themes:

1. Biophotons as the Missing Nutrient

- Cells emit and absorb photons during vital processes, including oxidative phosphorylation and DNA repair.
- A deficiency in biophotonic coherence underlies many modern disorders, from chronic fatigue to neurodegeneration.

2. Quantum Nutrition Defined

- Nutrition is reconceptualized as more than food. It includes sunlight, structured water, circadian alignment, breath, and consciousness.
- Biophoton-rich foods and natural rhythms replenish cellular order and resilience.

3. The Science of Coherence

- Coherence—the organized flow of light in biological systems—is presented as a universal biomarker of health.
- Disorders arise when coherence is lost. Healing occurs when light is restored.

4. Bridging Ancient Wisdom and Modern Biophysics

- Traditional healing systems (e.g., Ayurveda, Chinese medicine) described "qi" or "prana" as vital energy.
- Quantum biology now provides scientific language to validate these principles through biophoton research.

What Readers Will Gain:

By the end of Part I, readers will:

- Understand why light is life's most essential nutrient, shaping everything from mitochondrial energy to consciousness.
- Recognize how diet, lifestyle, and environment affect the body's light economy.
- Begin to see health and disease not as biochemical imbalances alone, but as patterns of light coherence or deficiency.

CHAPTER 1

What Is Biophoton Quantum Nutrition?

Redefining Food, Energy, and the Invisible Forces That Nourish Life

---

We are not only nourished by food, but by the light and information it carries.

—Fritz-Albert Popp, PhD

From Molecules to Light

For much of modern history, nutrition has been defined by what can be weighed and measured: calories, proteins, fats, carbohydrates, vitamins, and minerals. Food, in this framework, is primarily a fuel collection of molecules broken down to provide energy and raw materials for growth and repair. This biochemical model has been invaluable in treating nutrient deficiencies such as scurvy, rickets, and anemia.

Yet, this model overlooks a deeper layer of nourishment—one rooted not in matter, but in **energy, light, and information.**

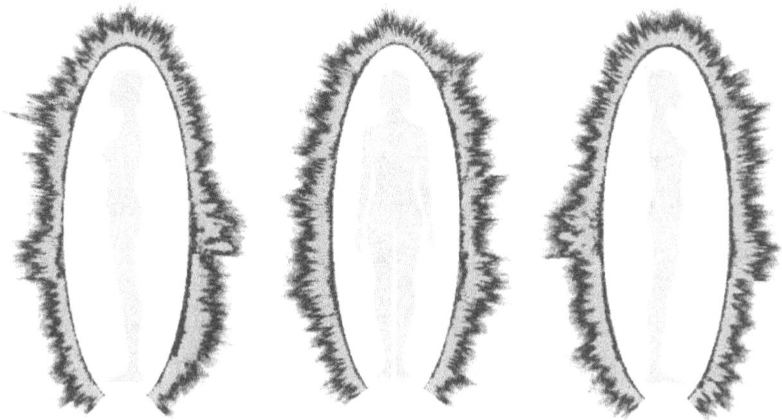

Figure 1.1. A Healthy Human Body Is Radiating Biophotons Naturally.
Visualization of the human biofield demonstrates that the human body is full of biophotons. The surrounding colorful emissions represent ultra-weak photon radiation naturally produced by living cells, highlighting the body's intrinsic light-based communication system.

Quantum nutrition extends beyond the boundaries of classical nutrition. It is built on the recognition that life is not sustained by chemistry alone, but also by a web of electromagnetic fields, photon emissions, and quantum coherence. Every cell is a quantum system:

- DNA emits ultra-weak photons detectable by sensitive instruments [1].
- Mitochondria respond directly to red and near-infrared light, altering ATP production [2].
- Enzymes rely on quantum tunneling to catalyze reactions essential for life [3].

Thus, food is not merely substance. It is a carrier of biological signals encoded in light frequencies, molecular vibrations, and electromagnetic patterns.

The Limits of Classical Nutrition

Traditional nutrition has excelled at treating deficiencies; however, new paradoxes have emerged in modern societies: people consume sufficient, or even excess, calories and micronutrients, yet still suffer from fatigue, chronic inflammation, metabolic diseases, and premature aging.

Why? Something beyond chemical composition is missing. Research shows that fresh, unprocessed foods emit biophotons, a form of ultra-weak light in the ultraviolet and visible spectrum [4,5]. These emissions are not random; they serve as regulatory signals within biological systems.

Fritz-Albert Popp demonstrated that the coherence of biophoton emissions correlates with biological vitality:

- Highly coherent emissions → organized, resilient systems.
- Chaotic or diminished emissions → disease and dysfunction [6,7].

This suggests that the "life force" of food is not simply its molecular content, but its light quality.

Defining Quantum Nutrition

Quantum nutrition is the science and practice of nourishing the human system by optimizing not only the material contents of food but also its energetic and informational dimensions.

It rests on three guiding principles:

1. Food as Energy and Information
   Each meal carries encoded biological signals transmitted through light, frequency, and structure.

2. The Body as a Quantum Field
   Cells and organs communicate through electromagnetic fields and photon emissions, generating coherence when healthy, and disharmony when diseased [8].
3. Nourishment as Multidimensional
   True nutrition includes molecules and vibrational resonance, electromagnetic harmony, and consciousness.

A New Framework: Beyond Calories and Chemistry

Category	Classical Nutrition	Quantum Nutrition
Core Basis	Molecules, calories, enzymes	Photons, frequencies, coherence
Primary Orientation	Focus on deficiency/excess	Focus on bioenergetic alignment
Measurement Approach	Measures quantity	Measures quality of light and information
Health Strategy	Reactive (treats disease)	Preventive and regenerative
Foundational Inputs	Based on material inputs	Based on energy, intention, and structure

Why Light Matters

Sunlight is humanity's first and most essential nutrient. Without it, photosynthesis—and therefore all food chains—would collapse. But light does more than sustain plants:

- It regulates circadian rhythms, hormones, and metabolism in humans [9–10].
- Within organisms, biophotons regulate DNA repair, cellular communication, and growth [11].
- A strong biophoton field is effective in treating many common diseases [14–24].

Foods grown in natural sunlight, harvested fresh, and consumed raw or gently cooked retain higher levels of coherent photon energy. By contrast, foods that are processed, irradiated, or chemically altered often show degraded photon emissions, even when vitamin and mineral levels remain intact [12–13].

Thus, Quantum nutrition places a premium on biophoton-rich foods, as these directly support the body's intrinsic light-based communication systems.

Quantum Nutrition in Practice

The principles of Biophoton Quantum Nutrition translate into simple, practical practices:

- Choose photon-rich foods: fresh greens, sprouts, wild berries [12,13].
- Avoid energetically "dead" foods: ultra-processed, microwaved, or irradiated items.
- Incorporate structured water and regular exposure to natural sunlight.
- Use intention and gratitude as amplifiers of nutritional coherence.

Toward a New Definition of Nourishment

Nutrition in the quantum age requires us to move beyond reductionist models and embrace a holistic, energetic, and integrative paradigm. Food is not only matter but also light, frequency, and consciousness.

To eat, then, is not simply to sustain the body; it is to align with the organizing intelligence of life itself.

This framework defines what we term Biophoton Quantum Nutrition: a new frontier of nourishment, rooted in ancient wisdom, validated by modern science, and essential for radiant health in the 21st century.

References

1. Popp FA, Gu Q, and Li KH. Biophoton emission: experimental background and theoretical approaches. *Modern Physics Letters B*. 1994;*8(21-22):1269-1296 (1994)*.

2. Hamblin MR. Shining light on the head: Photobiomodulation for brain disorders. *BBA Clin*. 2016 Oct 1(6):113-124. doi: 10.1016/j.bbacli.2016.09.002.

3. Ball P. Quantum biology: Better living through quantum mechanics. *Nature*. 2011;474:272–274.

4. van Wijk R, van Wijk EPA, Popp FA. Ultraweak photon emission: A tool for health and disease assessment. *J Photochem Photobiol B*. 2005;79(2):189–207.

5. Cifra M, Pospíšil P. Ultra-weak photon emission from biological samples: Definition, mechanisms, properties, detection and applications. *J Photochem Photobiol B*. 2014;139:2–10.

6. Popp FA, Nagl W, Li KH, et al. Biophoton emission: New evidence for coherence and DNA as source. *Cell Biophys*. 1984;6(1):33–52.

7. Popp FA, Beloussov LV, editors. *Integrative Biophysics: Biophotonics*. Dordrecht, Netherlands: Kluwer Academic Publishers; 2003.

8. Albrecht-Buehler G. Cellular infrared detector appears to be contained in the centrosome. *Cell Motil Cytoskeleton.* 1994;27(3):262–271.

9. Foster RG, Kreitzman L. *The rhythms of life: What your body clock means to you.* New Haven: Yale University Press; 2004.

10. Liu JZ, Gu HY. Biophotons reverse aging caused by circadian rhythm disruption. In: Younger by Light. Authors on Mission; 2025.

11. Popp FA, Chang JJ, Herzog A, et al. Evidence of non-classical (squeezed) light in biological systems. *Phys Lett A.* 2002;293(1–2):98–102.

12. van Wijk R. *Light in shaping life: Biophotons in biology and medicine.* Meluna; 2014.

13. Bajpai RP. Quantum coherence of biophotons and living systems. *Indian J Exp Biol.* 2003;41(5):514–527.

14. Liu JZ, Ramirez AD, Osborn K, Osborn L, Ager A, Gu HY. Biophoton quantum therapy enabled cancer treatments to reach their utmost goal of cancer-free. *Gerontol Geriatr Stud.* 2025;9(4):GGS.000718.

15. Tartak D, Gu HY, Robinson S, Silva I, Liu JL. Biophoton quantum therapy to treat advanced glaucoma: A novel non-invasive approach for ocular neuroprotection. *Biomed J Sci Tech Res.* 2025;62(3):BJSTR.MS.ID.009739.

16. Hu Y, Gu HY, Liu JZ. Reversal of tissue glycation and cholesterol accumulation by strong biophotons: A new anti-aging mechanism. *Gerontol Geriatr Stud.* 2025;9(3):GGS.000715. doi:10.31031/GGS.2025.09.000715

17. Liu JZ, Smotrys M, Robinson SD, Liu S, Gu HY. Therapeutic benefits of biophoton therapy in Parkinson's disease: Clinical evidence from a pilot and real-world study. *J Neurol Res Rev Rep.* 2025;7(6):1–6.

18. Liu JZ, Smotrys MA, Robinson SD, Yu HX, Liu SX, Liu DR, Gu HY. Multimodal evidence of cognitive restoration in Alzheimer's disease following biophoton therapy: A neurophysiological and energetic assessment. *SRC/JADR.* 2025;107. doi:10.47363/JADR/2025(2)107.

19. Liu JZ, Smotrys MA, Robinson SD, Yu HX, Liu SX, Liu DR, Gu HY. A breakthrough in stroke rehabilitation: Non-invasive biophoton therapy promotes neurofunctional recovery in chronic stroke patients. *SRC/JADR.* 2025;109.

CHAPTER 2

Quantum Nutrients

The Subtle Substances That Nourish Beyond Chemistry

We are more than matter. We are structured, vibrating light—and through light, we heal.

—James Z. Liu, MD, PhD

Beyond Biochemistry: The Rise of Quantum Nutrients

For centuries, nutrition was defined almost exclusively in chemical terms: carbohydrates, proteins, fats, vitamins, and minerals—quantified in calories, grams, and milligrams. This model explained much about energy balance and deficiency diseases. Yet, it fails to account for the energetic and informational dimensions of nourishment revealed by quantum biology, biophotonics, and biofield science [1–3].

Quantum nutrients are not defined solely by molecular weight or caloric density. Instead, they are distinguished by their vibrational energy, coherence, and informational signatures. These subtle properties interact with the biofield, the organizing energy field that surrounds and permeates the human body [6]. By influencing DNA expressions, mitochondrial dynamics, and intercellular communication, quantum nutrients help orchestrate vitality in ways often invisible to standard laboratory assays.

What Makes a Nutrient "Quantum"?

A quantum nutrient is any natural or technologically enhanced substance that nourishes life by delivering light, frequency, and coherence, rather than just biochemical mass. These substances act through:

- Biophoton emission: ultra-weak light emitted continuously by living cells [1,4,10].
- Electromagnetic frequency coherence: resonance patterns that synchronize biological processes [2].
- Molecular vibrational resonance: subtle oscillations influencing enzyme activity and signaling [3].
- Biofield interaction: restoring or strengthening coherence within the body's energy field [6].

Quantum nutrients are most abundant in fresh, wild, or minimally processed foods, structured water, and vibrational remedies. Unlike synthetic isolates, they synergize with the body's energy systems, amplifying self-repair, resilience, and even higher consciousness.

Quantum Nutrients in the Digestive Journey

To understand how these subtle properties shape human health, it is useful to trace how quantum nutrients move through the body:

Digestion

- Quantum-rich foods (e.g., sprouts, fruits, raw greens) not only break down into amino acids, sugars, and fatty acids but also release biophotonic energy that interacts with the gut biofield.
- The gut microbiome, an active biophotonic ecosystem, responds to coherent foods with improved microbial balance [7].

Absorption

- In the small intestine, structured water layers within villi enhance nutrient transport.
- Quantum nutrients, through vibrational resonance, facilitate more efficient cellular uptake, particularly in mitochondria-rich tissues [4,9].

Metabolism

- Once in circulation, mitochondria translate not only chemical fuels but also photonic and vibrational inputs into ATP [2,3].
- Coherent nutrients reduce oxidative stress, stabilize enzymatic reactions, and improve redox signaling.

Biological Function

- Quantum nutrients regulate gene expression, stem cell activity, and intercellular communication [1,5].
- They help synchronize circadian rhythms, hormone release, and nervous system coherence [6].

Excretion

- Foods lacking coherence (highly processed, irradiated, or chemically denatured) create metabolic "noise" and leave greater toxic residue.
- Quantum-rich nutrients minimize waste, as more of their informational content is used for repair and renewal.

Key Insight: Quantum nutrition enhances not only the quantity of absorbed nutrients but also the quality of biological communication that those nutrients enable.

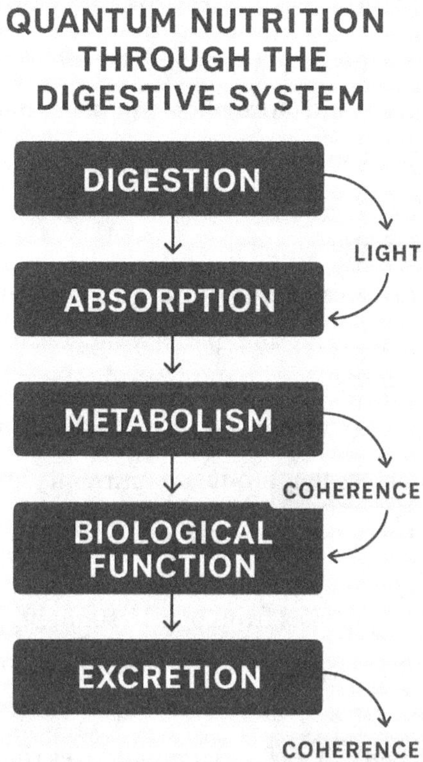

Figure 2.1. Quantum Nutrition Through the Digestive System. *This flowchart illustrates how quantum nutrition extends beyond classical biochemical digestion into energetic and informational processes. Ingestion of high-biophoton foods initiates digestion, where both molecular nutrients and biophotonic energy are released. During absorption, structured water and intestinal processes facilitate not only nutrient uptake but also the transfer of photon information into cells. Metabolism is powered by mitochondria, which utilize both substrates and light coherence to optimize ATP production. At the level of biological function, biophotons regulate DNA expression, hormonal balance, and intercellular communication through coherence. Finally, in excretion, low-coherence inputs leave waste, whereas high-coherence nutrition minimizes toxic residue, maintaining systemic alignment. Together, these stages highlight how light and coherence serve as critical regulators of human vitality alongside traditional biochemical pathways.*

Examples of Quantum Nutrients in Nature

- Sun-ripened fruits and vegetables
  Plants capture and store photons during photosynthesis. When eaten fresh, they deliver biophotons that support metabolic efficiency and cellular communication [5,10].
- Sprouts and microgreens
  Rich in life-force energy, these actively dividing cells offer potent regenerative and detoxifying effects.
- Medicinal mushrooms (e.g., reishi, lion's mane)
  Carry complex vibrational signatures and bioactive polysaccharides that modulate immunity and neural function [3].
- Raw honey
  Encodes frequencies from plants, sunlight, and bees, functioning as a vibrationally imprinted superfood.
- Structured spring water
  Forms hexagonal molecular geometries that more effectively store and transmit biological information [4,9].

Human-Enhanced Quantum Nutrients

Technological advances now allow us to amplify nature's blueprint:

- Biophoton-charged oils and minerals
  Encoded with structured light to promote cellular repair [1,5].
- Homeopathics and flower essences
  Chemically dilute but vibrationally potent, influencing subtle physiology and emotion [7].
- Tesla BioHealers and Biophoton Generators
  Emit coherent photonic fields that recharge mitochondria, support stem cell activity, and revitalize metabolism.

- Quantum-coded supplements
  Infused with frequencies such as Schumann resonance or solfeggio tones, harmonizing nervous and endocrine systems [8].

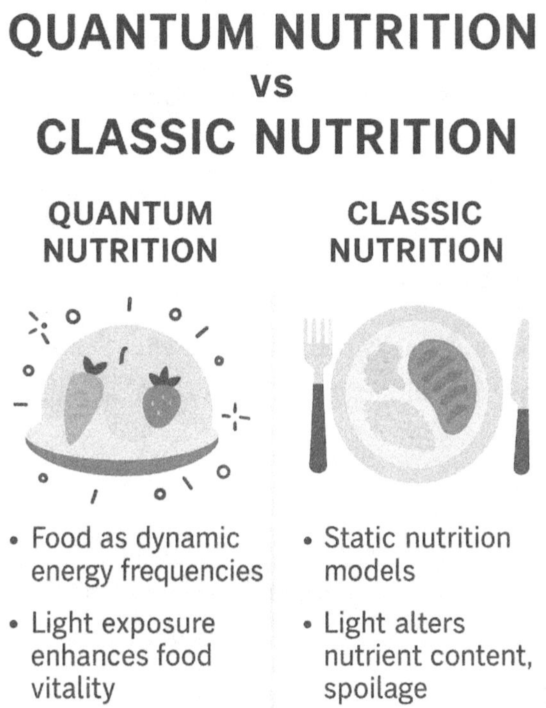

Figure 2.2. Quantum Nutrition vs. Classic Nutrition. *Quantum nutrition views food as dynamic energy frequencies enhanced by light exposure, while Classic Nutrition focuses on static nutrient models affected by light and spoilage.*

Why Quantum Nutrients Matter

Mitochondria, the central hubs of energy metabolism, respond not only to glucose, fatty acids, and oxygen but also to light and coherent vibrational signals [2,3]. Aging, fatigue, and chronic illness are increasingly viewed as disorders of communication and coherence within the biofield [6].

Quantum nutrients help restore this coherence. They act as informational inputs, teaching the body not only what to do but how to do it—efficiently, harmoniously, and in rhythm with biological cycles.

Toward a New Model of Nourishment

As bioenergetics and quantum biology expand, the definition of health is shifting from chemical sufficiency to energetic coherence. Quantum nutrients, once considered "alternative," will be recognized as foundational; essential for cellular vitality, regenerative capacity, and human flourishing [11–14].

Ultimately, we are not only matter. We are light encoded in structure, frequency, and form. And through that light, we heal.

Key Takeaway

Quantum nutrients nourish not only the body's biochemistry but also its energetic blueprint. They provide coherence, frequency, and light—subtle yet essential ingredients for vibrant health, longevity, and awakened consciousness.

References

1. Popp FA, et al. Biophoton emission: New evidence for coherence in living biological systems. In: *Electromagnetic Bio-Information.* Munich: Urban & Schwarzenberg. 1981;123–149.

2. van Wijk R, van Wijk EPA. Biophotons and bio-communication. *J Sci Explor.* 2005;19(4):531–545.

3. Bischof M. Biophotons– The light in our cells. *J Optometric Phototherapy*. 2005;13(1):2–6.

4. Del Giudice E, Tedeschi A. Water and autocatalysis in living matter. *Electromagn Biol Med.* 2009;28(1):46–52.

5. Tiller WA. *Science and human transformation: Subtle energies, intentionality and consciousness.* Pavior Publishing; 1997.

6. Chen L, Michalsen A. Management of chronic pain using complementary and integrative medicine. *BMJ* 2017;357:j1284.

7. Krasnoholovets V. *Submicroscopic deterministic quantum mechanics.* Ukrainian Academy of Sciences; 2004.

8. Pollack GH. *The fourth phase of water: Beyond solid, liquid, and vapor.* Ebner & Sons; 2013.

9. Fels D. Cellular communication through light. *PLoS One.* 2009;4(4):e5086.

10. Liu JZ, Gu HY, and Liu DR. Biophoton generators enhance germination, preserve produce and boost fermentation: A new frontier in quantum nutrition and agriculture. *Nov Tech Nutri Food Sci.* 2025;8(4). NTNF. 000691. doi:10.31031/NTNF.2025.08.000691.

11. Smotrys MA, Liu JZ, Street S., and Robinson S. Energetic homeostasis achieved through biophoton energy and accompanying medication treatment resulted in sustained levels of thyroiditis-Hashimoto's, iron, vitamin D & vitamin B12. *Metabolism Open. 2023;*18:100248.

12. Liu JZ, Poirier L, Louie J, Gu HY. Non-Invasive biophoton therapy restores visual function in advanced glaucoma: A human and canine case report. *Journal of Neurology Research*

Reviews & Reports. SRC/JNRRR. 2025;289. doi:10.47363/JNRRR/2025(7)231.

13. Liu JZ, Smotrys MA, Robinson SD, Yu HX, Liu SX, Liu DR, and Gu HY. Biophoton therapy in Lyme Disease: Neurophysiological and bioenergetic improvements over 4 weeks - A case report. *Journal of Neurology Research Reviews & Reports. SRC/JNRRR.* 2025;292.

CHAPTER 3

The Biophysics of Life

Quantum Fields, Coherence, and Bioenergetics

The body is not a machine made of matter—it is a field of energy, frequency, and vibration.

—Nikola Tesla (paraphrased)

Beyond the Mechanical Body

Nutrition is not merely about fueling a biochemical machine; it is about nourishing a living, vibrating system of quantum fields and light. Classical physiology views the body as a collection of organs and chemical reactions, but quantum biology reveals it as an electromagnetic matrix, regulated by coherence, resonance, and light-based signaling [1,2].

To grasp quantum nutrition, we must first understand the biophysical foundation of life.

The Body as a Quantum Energy System

At its core, the human body functions as a coherent quantum system [3]. Every cell is both a biochemical entity and an electromagnetic oscillator, surrounded by and embedded in biofields. These fields are not accidental byproducts; they are essential regulators of growth, repair, and communication.

Key features of the body as a quantum system include:

- Coherence: Waves and photons vibrating in synchrony; coherence in biology reflects harmonious cell-to-cell communication [1,4].
- Nonlocality: Biological systems demonstrate long-range correlations, suggesting energetic entanglement across tissues [5].
- Quantum tunneling: Enzymes exploit quantum tunneling to transfer electrons across energy barriers, explaining catalytic speeds beyond classical limits [6].

Together, these phenomena point to a level of bioenergetic regulation deeper than chemistry alone.

Coherence: The Music of Health

Coherence in biology can be compared to a symphony. When all instruments play in tune, the music resonates beautifully. In health, coherent biophoton emissions serve as this harmony.

Fritz-Albert Popp's pioneering research demonstrated that:

- Healthy cells emit coherent light to maintain communication.
- Cancerous or stressed cells emit chaotic or excessive photons.
- Biophoton signals encode the informational structure of life itself [1,7].

When nutrition supports coherence, the body naturally shifts toward self-regulation, repair, and vitality.

The Role of Electromagnetic Fields in Biology

Every cell generates and responds to electromagnetic fields:

- The membrane potential controls ion gradients critical for signaling.

- Cells use oscillations and field effects for tissue coordination.
- External frequencies—light, sound, and magnetic fields—can influence growth and repair [2,8].

Evidence shows that electromagnetic cues help regulate embryonic development, wound healing, and regeneration [9]. This explains why disruptive EMFs (e.g., Wi-Fi, phones) can interfere with physiology, while therapeutic fields (pulsed EMFs, infrared light) promote healing [10].

The Biofield: The Body's Master Energy System

Surrounding and permeating the body is the biofield, an organized energy system now recognized in medical research [11].

Functions of the biofield include:

- Regulating growth, repair, and immune responses.
- Storing informational blueprints for optimal health.
- Acting as an interface between consciousness, nutrition, and physiology [12].

Quantum nutrition supports the biofield by providing coherent frequencies, photonic energy, and vibrational foods.

Mitochondria: Bioenergetic Power Plants That Respond to Light

Mitochondria are well known for producing ATP, but recent studies reveal additional roles:

- They act as photoreceptors, responding especially to red and near-infrared light [13].
- They regulate apoptosis, calcium homeostasis, and stem cell activation.

- They both emit and absorb biophotons, contributing to cellular communication networks [14].

Thus, mitochondria can be fueled not only by B vitamins or CoQ10, but also by light inputs from sunlight or high-photon foods. Mitochondrion in a coherent photonic environment is more efficient and resilient.

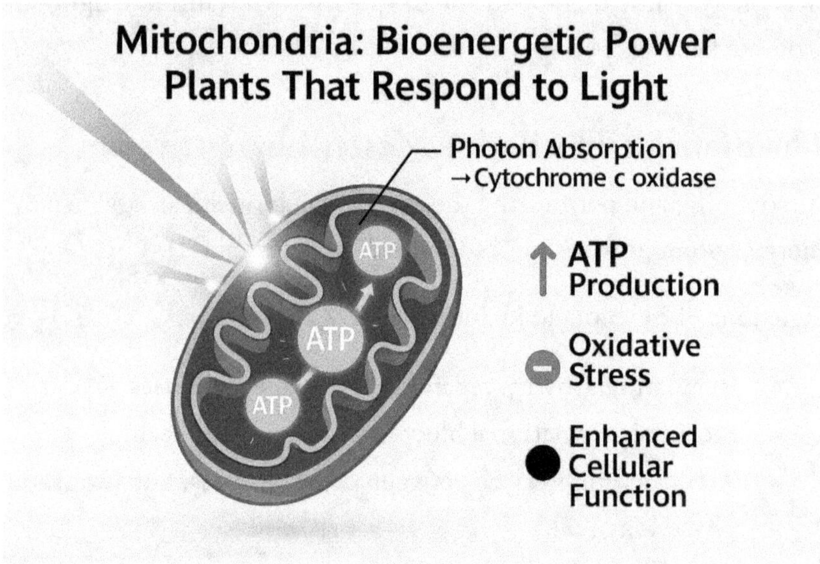

Figure 3.1. Mitochondria: Bioenergetic Power Plants That Respond to Light. *Mitochondria are bioenergetic power plants that respond to light. Biophotons absorbed by cytochrome c oxidase stimulate increased ATP production, reduce oxidative stress, and enhance overall cellular function.*

Structured Water: The Hidden Medium of Bioelectricity

Water inside cells is not ordinary liquid but exists, in part, in a structured "fourth phase" (exclusion zone, EZ) [15]. Structured water:

- Aligns along proteins and membranes.
- Stores energy from sunlight and biophotons.

- Functions as a liquid crystal, supporting charge separation and information storage [15,16].

Pollack's work shows that EZ water acts like a biological battery, charged by infrared light [15]. Foods like cucumbers, aloe, and spring water, along with natural sunlight, enhance cellular water structuring.

Food as Electromagnetic Input

Beyond calories, every food carries a vibrational signature that influences the body's field.

- Leafy greens: rich in photons that support immune and cardiovascular coherence.
- Fermented foods: emit organized electromagnetic patterns that regulate gut-brain communication.
- Fresh fruits: high in light content and frequency patterns resonant with mitochondrial pathways.

By contrast, processed and irradiated foods emit depleted or chaotic signals, introducing energetic noise [3,7].

Consciousness: The Most Subtle Nutrient

Perhaps the most overlooked element of nutrition is consciousness itself. The act of eating is not merely physical; it is influenced by intention, gratitude, and observation. Quantum physics demonstrates that the observer influences outcomes, and biology reflects the same principle [5].

Emotional state during eating can affect digestion, absorption, and even biophoton emissions [12]. Thus, conscious presence is itself a nutrient.

Summary: The Quantum Body Demands Quantum Nourishment

Biophysical System	Nutritional Influence
Biophoton emission	Supported by fresh, light-rich foods
Coherent EM fields	Enhanced by grounding, structured water, and sunlight
Mitochondria	Energized by red/infrared light and raw produce
Structured water	Promoted by hydrating foods and infrared
Biofield integrity	Strengthened by intention, harmony, and vibrational foods

Understanding the biophysics of life is the foundation for quantum nutrition. It shows us that food, light, water, and intention are all parts of a unified energy ecology. In the next chapter, we turn to biophotons, the luminous messengers of cellular vitality, that bridge quantum science and nutrition.

References

1. Popp FA, et al. Biophoton emission: New evidence for coherence in living systems. Electromagn Bio-Information. Urban & Schwarzenberg; 1981.

2. van Wijk R. Light in Shaping Life: Biophotons in Biology and Medicine. Meluna Publishing; 2014.

3. Bischof M. Biophotons – The Light in Our Cells. J Optometric Phototherapy. 2005;13(1):2–6.

4. Bajpai RP. Quantum coherence of biophotons and living systems. Indian J Exp Biol. 2003;41(5):514–527.

5. Fels D. Cellular communication through light. PLoS One. 2009;4(4):e5086. doi:10.1371/journal.pone.0005086

6. Ball P. Quantum biology: Better living through quantum mechanics. Nature. 2011;474:272–274.

7. Popp FA, Chang JJ, Herzog A, et al. Evidence of non-classical (squeezed) light in biological systems. Phys Lett A. 2002;293(1-2):98–102.

8. Adey WR. Biological effects of electromagnetic fields. J Cell Biochem. 1993;51(4):410–416.

9. Levin M. Reprogramming cells and tissue patterning via bioelectrical pathways: molecular mechanisms and biomedical opportunities. Wiley Interdiscip Rev Syst Biol Med. 2013 Nov-Dec;5(6):657-76. doi: 10.1002/wsbm.1236. Epub 2013 Jul 29.

10. Shen Q. Gu H. and Yan Y. Photobiomodulation for neurodegenerative diseases: A scoping review. Int J Mol Sci. 2024 Jan 28;25(3):1625.

11. Trivedi MK et al. The use of biofield energy therapy as complementary and alternative medicine in the human health care system: a narrative review and potential mechanisms. J Complement Integr Med. 2024 Apr 3;21(4):451–460.

12. Rubik B. The biofield hypothesis: Its biophysical basis and role in medicine. J Altern Complement Med. 2002;8(6):703–717. doi:10.1089/10755530260511711.

13. Wong-Riley MTT, et al. Photobiomodulation directly benefits primary neurons functionally inactivated by toxins. J Biol Chem. 2005;280(6):4761–4771.

14. Tang, R. and Dai, J. Biophoton signal transmission and processing in the brain. Journal of Photochemistry and Photobiology B. 2014;139: 71-75.

15. Pollack GH. The fourth phase of water: Beyond solid, liquid, and vapor. Ebner & Sons; 2013.

16. Del Giudice E, Tedeschi A. Water and autocatalysis in living matter. Electromagn Biol Med. 2009;28(1):46–52.

CHAPTER 4

Biophotons—Light Within Living Cells

The Missing Nutrient at the Quantum Level

We know today that man is essentially a being of light.
—Fritz-Albert Popp, PhD

Biophotons: The Quantum Messengers of Life

If quantum nutrition has a central messenger, it is the biophoton. Invisible to the naked eye yet measurable by ultrasensitive detectors, biophotons are ultraweak light emissions in the ultraviolet to visible spectrum, continuously radiated by all living organisms [1,2].

Far from being biochemical curiosities, biophotons play regulatory and organizational roles in biology. They may be the "missing nutrient" in human health—a subtle but essential input that sustains coherence, vitality, and communication across the body.

What Are Biophotons?

Biophotons are light particles emitted spontaneously by living systems, originating mainly from DNA, mitochondria, and cellular membranes [1]. First observed in the 1920s and rigorously investigated by Fritz-Albert Popp in the 1970s, they were shown to be emitted not randomly but with coherence, a property in which photons oscillate in synchrony, much like laser light [2,3].

This coherence suggests that biophotons are not byproducts of metabolism but rather functional signals used to regulate order and harmony in living systems [4].

Functions of Biophotons in Biology

1. Cellular Communication

- Travel faster than chemical messengers.
- Use DNA and microtubules as "light waveguides" to transmit information [5].
- Synchronize mitosis, repair, and stress responses across tissues.

2. Genetic Regulation

- DNA acts as both an emitter and receiver of light [6].
- Photonic interactions influence gene expression, epigenetic switches, and DNA repair.
- The physical twist and shape of DNA modulate photon emission patterns.

3. Metabolic Efficiency

- Mitochondria respond to red and near-infrared light by increasing ATP output [7].
- Biophotonic coherence minimizes entropy, making enzymatic reactions more efficient [8].

4. Health Assessment

- Cancerous and inflamed cells show chaotic or excessive photon bursts.
- Healthy cells emit low-intensity, rhythmic, ordered pulses [2,9].

- Photon emission patterns may one day be used for non-invasive diagnostics.

Food as a Source of Biophotons

Popp's studies demonstrated that foods differ dramatically in their photon emissions [3]:

- Fresh, organic, sun-ripened produce has the highest levels of coherent light.
- Processed, irradiated, or microwaved foods show degraded or chaotic emissions.
- The "aliveness" of food is reflected in its photon output and its ability to restore coherence to the human system [2].

In this sense, biophotons in food act as informational nutrients, helping the body re-establish its natural order.

Measuring Biophoton Activity

Biophotons can be measured using photomultiplier tubes (PMTs) and ultrasensitive CCD cameras [1]. Applications include:

- Food vitality testing: ranking produce by photon output.
- Disease monitoring: tracking coherence shifts during stress, healing, or degeneration [9].
- Water studies: comparing photon storage and release in structured vs. unstructured water [10].

Emerging imaging techniques now allow visualization of photon emissions from hands, plants, and microbes, revealing the light language of life.

Biophoton Deficiency: A Modern Mal-Illumination

If biophotons are essential nutrients, modern lifestyles create a deficiency. Contributing factors include:

- Reliance on processed, low-light foods.
- Artificial lighting with little full-spectrum input.
- Limited natural sunlight exposure.
- Electromagnetic pollution disrupts coherence [11].
- Mitochondrial dysfunction reduces photon output.

The result is what Popp called "mal-illumination"—low vitality, poor regeneration, brain fog, inflammation, and accelerated aging [3]. Quantum nutrition seeks to reverse this by restoring light-rich food, sunlight, and coherent photonic environments.

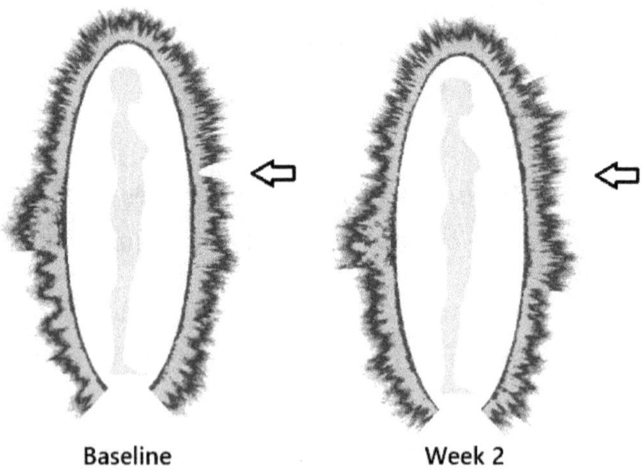

Figure 4.1. Biophoton Coherence Before and After Treatment. *Gas discharge visualization (GDV) imaging of the human biofield at Baseline (left) compared to Week 2 after biophoton treatment (right). At baseline, the aura appears fragmented with irregular gaps, indicating reduced coherence and weakened energy distribution. After two weeks of biophoton exposure, the biofield shows greater symmetry, brightness, and uniformity, reflecting improved biophoton coherence and systemic vitality.*

Lessons from the Animal Kingdom

In nature, survival is linked to biophoton intake.

- Large predators thrive on the fresh meat of recently living animals—still rich in coherent photon energy.
- Herbivores flourish by consuming sunlight-infused plants.

Both strategies rely on accessing fresh, biophoton-rich sources of nutrition, underscoring light's role as a driver of biological vitality.

Practical Ways to Increase Biophoton Intake

Practice	Biophoton Impact
Eat raw, organic, sun-ripened fruits and greens.	Supplies coherent light frequencies
Avoid microwaved/irradiated foods.	Prevents chaotic emissions
Drink structured or spring water.	Enhances photon storage and transfer [10]
Get daily morning sunlight.	Recharges mitochondria and skin photoreceptors [7]
Use biophoton-enhancing technologies (e.g., Tesla BioHealers, red-light therapy).	Amplifies ambient coherence
Practice gratitude and mindfulness at meals.	Strengthens biofield and digestion [12]

Biophotons as Quantum Nutrients

By the classical definition, nutrients are essential for growth, repair, and survival. Biophotons, though not made of atoms, fulfill this role:

- They are essential for optimal cellular function.

- They are absorbed and emitted by tissues.
- Their absence correlates with dysfunction and disease.
- They can be supplemented through food, sunlight, and photonic technologies.

Thus, under the quantum nutrition paradigm, biophotons are real, functional nutrients.

Conclusion: Feed the Light, Become the Light

Your body is not just a biochemical machine—it is a living light field. Every meal is not only matter consumed but light absorbed and information encoded. Biophotons form the bridge between nutrition, consciousness, and vitality.

To nourish the body deeply is to feed your inner light, awakening the highest potential for healing, resilience, and evolution.

The next chapter will explore the biofield, the electromagnetic matrix that surrounds and informs the body, and how quantum nutrition strengthens this field to influence immunity, regeneration, and emotional balance.

References

1. Popp FA, et al. Biophoton emission: New evidence for coherence in living biological systems. Electromagn Bio-Information. Urban & Schwarzenberg; 1981.

2. van Wijk R, van Wijk EPA. Biophotons and bio-communication. J Sci Explor. 2005;19(4):531–545.

3. Popp FA, Beloussov LV. Integrative biophysics: Biophotonics. Springer; 2003.

4. Bajpai RP. Quantum coherence of biophotons and living systems. Indian J Exp Biol. 2003;41(5):514–527.

5. Tang R, Dai J. Biophoton signal transmission and biological information communication. Sci China C Life Sci. 2014;57(4):343–355.

6. Popp FA, Chang JJ, Herzog A, et al. Evidence of non-classical light in biological systems. Phys Lett A. 2002;293(1–2):98–102.

7. Hamblin MR. Shining light on the head: Photobiomodulation for brain disorders. BBA Clin 2016 Oct 1:6:113-124.

8. Ball P. Quantum biology: Better living through quantum mechanics. Nature. 2011;474:272–274.

9. Scholkmann F, et al. Ultraweak photon emission as a non-invasive health assessment method. J Photochem Photobiol B. 2013;139:2–10.

10. Del Giudice E, Tedeschi A. Water and autocatalysis in living matter. Electromagn Biol Med. 2009;28(1):46–52.

11. Adey WR. Biological effects of electromagnetic fields. J Cell Biochem. 1993;51(4):410–416.

12. Rubik B. The biofield hypothesis: Its biophysical basis and role in medicine. J Altern Complement Med. 2002;8(6):703–717.

CHAPTER 5

The Biofield and Nutritional Resonance

How the Body Interacts with Energy, Frequency, and Vibrational Nourishment

---

The field is the sole governing agency of the particle.
—Albert Einstein

Beyond Molecules: Nutrition as an Energetic Process

Most people imagine nutrition as molecules carried through the bloodstream to cells. While this is true biochemically, it is only part of the story. A deeper layer exists—an electromagnetic blueprint that both surrounds and penetrates the body. This biofield not only organizes physiology but also determines how food, water, light, and even emotions are received and metabolized [1,2].

In quantum nutrition, the biofield becomes central, regulating digestion, cellular communication, immune function, and consciousness itself. Fresh foods, coherent water, sunlight, and positive emotions all enhance the biofield, while processed food, chaotic environments, and stress degrade it.

What Is the Biofield?

The biofield is a dynamic, structured electromagnetic field generated by all living systems. The term was formally introduced in a 1994 NIH report to describe the ensemble of measurable electric, magnetic, photonic, and subtle fields that regulate biology [3].

The biofield includes:

- Electric fields from membrane potentials and ion channels.
- Magnetic fields from the brain, heart, and nerve activity (e.g., measured via MEG and ECG).
- Photonic fields (i.e., coherent light emissions from biophotons) [4].
- Subtle fields (scalar/torsion) are proposed to carry intention and nonlocal information [5].

Together, these layers form a holographic map of health. Disturbances in the biofield often precede symptoms of disease, while restoring coherence frequently precedes recovery [6].

Resonance: The Language of the Biofield

In physics, resonance occurs when two systems oscillate at the same frequency, amplifying energy transfer. In biology, resonance allows the body to:

- Recognize and integrate beneficial substances (nutrients, enzymes, photons).
- Repel or neutralize harmful inputs (toxins, pathogens).
- Synchronize tissues for regeneration and immune response [7].

Every meal, then, is not only chemical ingestion but also a resonance event: your biofield interacts with the vibrational frequency of the food. When frequencies match, harmony and vitality follow. When they clash, friction and inflammation may result.

How the Biofield Interacts with Nutrition

1. Biophoton-Rich Foods

- Emit coherent light that entrains the body toward order.
- Support mitochondrial signaling and cellular communication [4,8].
- Restore field coherence after stress.

2. Biophoton Technologies

- Devices such as coherent light generators or Tesla BioHealers amplify ambient photonic order.
- Rapidly restore resonance in disrupted biofields [9].

3. Structured Water

- Organizes into lattice-like arrays that store vibrational data [10].
- Acts as a conductor between biochemical reactions and bioelectrical networks.
- Enhances detoxification and nutrient transport.

4. Minerals and Trace Elements

- Carry natural electromagnetic charges.
- Stabilize membrane polarity and ion flow.
- Magnesium, zinc, and copper are essential for EM stability [11].

5. Emotionally Charged Eating

- Emotions emit measurable EM signatures (HRV, EEG).
- Gratitude and mindfulness create coherence; fear or anger fragments the field [12].
- Consciousness thus alters how nutrients are assimilated.

Assessing Biofield Health

Modern tools can now visualize and quantify aspects of the biofield:

Tool	Measurement
GDV (Gas Discharge Visualization)	Photon emission from fingertips, correlating with organ activity [13].
HRV (Heart Rate Variability)	Heart-brain coherence and systemic field alignment.
EIS (Electrointerstitial Scan)	Electrical conductivity along meridians.
Kirlian Photography	High-frequency emissions from skin surfaces.

Such tools are being integrated into energy medicine, biofeedback, and personalized nutrition, offering a window into vibrational health.

Restoring Nutritional Resonance

To optimize the biofield, one must restore coherence through resonant inputs:

- Eat whole, vibrant foods: Sun-ripened, organic foods carry stronger electromagnetic fields.
- Use biophoton and frequency therapies: PEMF, red light, and coherent field devices help "tune" the biofield.
- Practice mindful rituals: Gratitude, breathwork, and presence align the field with food.
- Cleanse your environment: Minimize EMF pollution, synthetic lighting, and chemical exposures.

Case Example

A 62-year-old woman with chronic fatigue had normal biochemical labs but poor biofield coherence, especially in her digestive region. Her diet was organic but heavily microwaved and eaten under fluorescent lights. After two weeks of switching to raw produce, structured water, biophoton-generator exposure, and gratitude practice before meals, her coherence improved—and her fatigue resolved. Her healing came not from chemistry, but from resonance restoration.

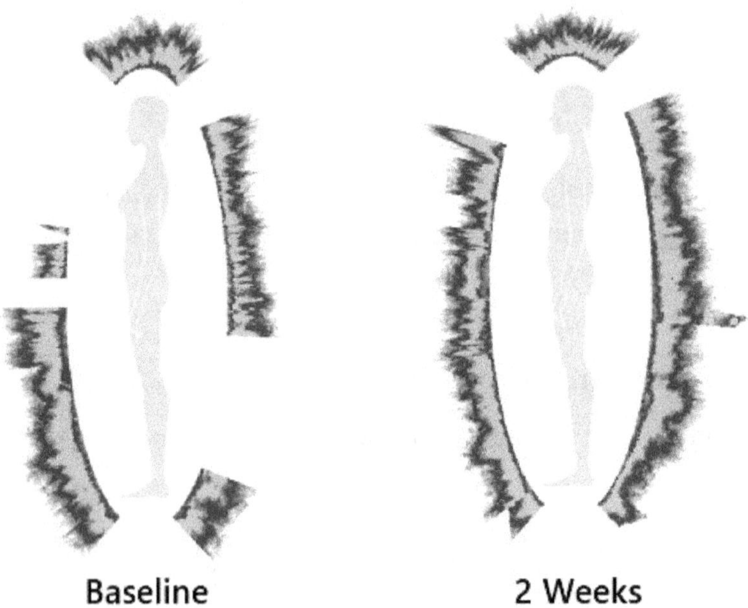

Figure 5.1. Improvement in Biophoton Coherence After Two Weeks of Treatment. *Gas discharge visualization (GDV) images of the human biofield at baseline (left) and after two weeks of biophoton treatment (right). At baseline, the biofield appears fragmented and discontinuous, with multiple gaps and irregularities reflecting reduced coherence and energetic imbalance. After two weeks of biophoton exposure, the biofield becomes more continuous, symmetric, and vibrant, indicating enhanced coherence, systemic alignment, and improved energetic vitality.*

Consciousness: The Hidden Variable

Quantum field theory and biofield science converge on one principle: consciousness influences matter.

- Thoughts and intentions affect how nutrients are received [5].
- Mindful eating entrains the heart, brain, and gut into coherence.
- Conscious rituals (e.g., blessing food) alter the vibrational structure of water and food, as shown in Emoto's crystallography experiments [14].

Thus, you don't just digest food, you co-create its meaning and effect.

Summary: Nourishing the Field Nourishes the Body

Biofield Principle	Nutritional Implication
Coherence = Health	Eat photon-rich, whole foods to maintain order.
Resonance guides assimilation	Choose foods/environments that match the body's frequency.
Structured energy = Absorbable energy	Use light, water, and intention to enhance availability.
Consciousness modulates outcome	Mindful eating transforms food into healing energy.

Quantum nutrition is biofield-centered nutrition. By restoring vibrational harmony, it feeds not only the cells but the very field of life that organizes them.

The next chapter explores how food carries quantum information, and how decoding this subtle information may help us reclaim resilience, vitality, and longevity.

References

1. Rubik B. The biofield hypothesis: Its biophysical basis and role in medicine. *J Altern Complement Med.* 2002;8(6):703–717.

2. Van Wijk R. *Light in shaping life: Biophotons in biology and medicine.* Meluna Publishing; 2014.

3. National Institutes of Health. Alternative medicine: Expanding medical horizons. *NIH Publication* 1994;94–066.

4. Popp FA, Beloussov LV. *Integrative biophysics: Biophotonics.* Springer; 2003.

5. Tiller WA. *Science and human transformation: Subtle energies, intentionality and consciousness.* Pavior Publishing; 1997.

6. Oschman JL. *Energy medicine: The scientific basis.* Churchill Livingstone; 2015.

7. Bajpai RP. Quantum coherence of biophotons and living systems. *Indian J Exp Biol.* 2003;41(5):514–527.

8. Fels D. Cellular communication through light. *PLoS One.* 2009;4(4):e5086.

9. Scholkmann F, et al. Ultraweak photon emission as a non-invasive health assessment method. *J Photochem Photobiol B.* 2013;139:2–10.

10. Pollack GH. *The fourth phase of water.* Ebner & Sons; 2013.

11. Athenstaedt H. Magnetic properties of biological systems. *J Biol Phys.* 1990;18(1):1–20.

12. McCraty R, Childre D. *Coherence: Bridging personal, social, and global health.* HeartMath Institute; 2010.

13. Korotkov KG. *Human energy field: Study with GDV bioelectrography.* Backbone Publishing; 2002.

14. Emoto M. *The hidden messages in water.* Beyond Words Publishing; 2004.

CHAPTER 6

Academic Teaching—Biophoton Quantum Nutrition

Educating the Next Generation of Light-Based Health Leaders

To teach quantum nutrition is to awaken students to the reality that food is not only matter but memory, frequency, and light. —**James Z. Liu, MD, PhD**

Introduction: Why Academic Teaching Matters

For quantum nutrition to reach its full potential, it must be integrated into education. Universities, medical schools, and nutrition programs continue to emphasize calories, macronutrients, and biochemistry, while neglecting the energetic and photonic dimensions of life. This knowledge gap leaves future clinicians, dietitians, and researchers unprepared to address chronic disease, aging, and ecological health through the lens of biophoton science.

Academic teaching of Biophoton Quantum Nutrition (BQN) ensures that the next generation of practitioners understands that:

- Cells communicate with photons, not just molecules [1,2].
- Nutritional value includes coherence and vitality, not just chemical content [3,4].
- Food systems must integrate sustainability and photonic health.
- Medicine can evolve from treating symptoms → restoring coherence.

Core Learning Objectives

An academic curriculum in BQN should prepare students to:

1. Understand the science of biophotons: origins, measurement, and role in biology.
2. Evaluate food quality based on light emission, coherence, and vitality.
3. Design nutritional interventions that include structured water, coherent foods, and biophotonic therapies.
4. Apply quantum principles in public health, agriculture, and clinical practice.
5. Critically assess research linking light, nutrition, and health outcomes.

Figure 6.1. Representation of a Healthy Human Biofield. *The image illustrates a human silhouette radiating a strong, coherent, and symmetrical golden aura, symbolizing optimal biophoton emission and biofield integrity. A balanced and expansive biofield reflects cellular vitality, mitochondrial efficiency, and systemic coherence, all of which are associated with resilience, health, and overall well-being.*

Curriculum Outline for Biophoton Quantum Nutrition

Module	Focus	Key Topics	Practical Application
1. Foundations of Biophotonics	Physics and biology of light in living systems	Ultraweak photon emission (UPE), DNA as a light source, mitochondrial photonics [1,2]	Lab demos with photomultiplier devices
2. Food as Light	Nutritional biophysics	Biophoton-rich foods, structured water, enzyme vitality [3,5]	Food quality testing, raw vs. processed
3. Quantum Nutrition and Human Health	Clinical perspectives	Biophoton deficiency in chronic disease, circadian nutrition, coherence-based diets [4,6]	Case studies of patients using BQN
4. Biophoton Agriculture	Farming and food systems	Light-based cultivation, reduced agrochemicals, sustainability [7,8]	Field projects, sprouting experiments
5. Clinical Biophoton Applications	Medicine and therapy	Red/NIR therapy, Tesla BioHealers, biofield medicine [6,9]	Practicum with biophoton devices
6. Research and Future Directions	Integrative science	AI, frequency mapping, global health impact [10]	Capstone research project

Teaching Strategies

- Interdisciplinary Approach: Integrating physics, biology, nutrition, and consciousness studies.
- Experiential Learning: Students measure biophoton emissions from fresh vs. processed foods.
- Case-Based Education: Analyzing patient and agricultural case studies where BQN improved outcomes.
- Technology Integration: Using GDV imaging, photomultiplier tubes, and structured water analysis in labs.
- Ethical and Ecological Discussions: Exploring how teaching light-based nutrition intersects sustainability and global food justice.

Academic Outcomes and Impact

Graduates trained in BQN will be positioned to:

- Pioneer quantum nutrition clinics that focus on coherence-based health care.
- Advise agricultural systems on light-enhanced cultivation and preservation.
- Advance research on chronic disease and aging through biophoton interventions.
- Influence policy and education, shaping how societies define nutrition in the 21st century.

Key Insight: Students exposed to quantum nutrition frameworks develop not only scientific literacy but also field awareness: the ability to sense coherence in food, environment, and human health.

Case Example: Classroom Demonstration

In one university course, students compared lettuce samples:

- Conventional supermarket lettuce (refrigerated, shipped long distances).
- Locally grown organic lettuce.
- Lettuce sprouted indoors in a biophoton-enhanced environment.

Using GDV imaging and photon counting, the third group displayed significantly stronger light emissions, which correlated with better flavor, freshness, and nutritional density. The experiment made a lasting impression, shifting student perspectives from "food as calories" to "food as light."

Summary: Building a New Paradigm in Education

Biophoton Quantum Nutrition belongs in every classroom where health, biology, or sustainability is taught.

Old Education Model	Quantum Nutrition Model
Calories, macronutrients	Light, frequency, coherence
Food as fuel	Food as information and intelligence
Disease prevention	Healthspan extension and coherence restoration
Linear science	Integrative, field-based science

To educate future leaders in health, agriculture, and medicine, we must teach the language of light.

References

1. Popp FA, Gu Q, and Li KH. Biophoton emission: Experimental background and theoretical approaches. *Modern Physics Letters B.* 1994;8(21-22):1272–1274.

2. Van Wijk R, Van Wijk EPA. Biophoton communication and regulation in living systems. *J Photochem Photobiol B.* 2005;79(2):141–147.

3. Bischof M. *Biophotons – The light in our cells.* Springer; 2008.

4. Pollack GH. *The fourth phase of water.* Ebner & Sons; 2013.

5. Hamblin MR. Mechanisms and Mitochondrial Redox Signaling in Photobiomodulation. *Photochemistry and Photobiology.* 94(2):199–212.

6. Ilic ZS. Light quality manipulation improves vegetable quality at harvest and postharvest: A review. *Environmental and Experimental Botany.* July 2017;139(special issue 1):79–90.

7. Musumeci F, et al. Coherence and electromagnetic order in plant development. *Bioelectromagnetics.* 2011;32(6):420–430.

8. Rubik B. The biofield hypothesis: its biophysical basis and role in medicine. *J Altern Complement Med.* 2002;8(6):703–717.

9. Salehpour F, Cassano P. Transcranial photobiomodulation therapy for cognition and mood. *Neurophotonics.* 2021;8(2):022001.

CHAPTER 7

Scientific Research in Biophoton Quantum Nutrition

Evidence, Experiments, and Emerging Directions

The future of nutrition will not be measured only in grams or calories, but in photons, coherence, and quantum order.

—James Z. Liu, MD, PhD

Introduction: From Hypothesis to Evidence

Quantum nutrition is more than a philosophical framework; it is a rapidly evolving scientific field grounded in biophoton research, photobiomodulation, and biofield studies. While conventional nutrition measures the chemical composition of food, biophoton research investigates how food emits, stores, and transfers light, and how these light-based signals regulate cellular processes.

Over the past four decades, pioneering studies have demonstrated that:

- All living systems emit ultraweak photon emissions (UPE) that correlate with metabolic and genetic activity [1,2].
- Food freshness and vitality can be quantified by its biophoton emission [3].
- Red and near-infrared light stimulate mitochondrial metabolism, confirming the role of photons in energy regulation [4].

- Quantum coherence is a unifying principle of biological health [5].

Key Insight: Scientific research indicates that many chronic conditions—such as fatigue, inflammation, and neurodegeneration—may not only reflect biochemical imbalances but also biophoton deficiency and incoherence.

Historical Foundations of Biophoton Science

- Alexander Gurwitsch (1920s): Discovered *mitogenetic radiation*—ultraviolet emissions from onion roots influencing cell division [6].
- Fritz-Albert Popp (1970s–2000s): Demonstrated that DNA emits highly coherent biophotons, theorizing that this coherence regulates biological communication and health [1].
- Van Wijk & Van Wijk (2005): Extended Popp's work to show that biophoton communication plays a role in systemic regulation [2].
- Pollack (2013): Demonstrated that water near hydrophilic surfaces stores radiant energy, forming *structured water (EZ water)* critical to bioenergetics [7].

These discoveries laid the foundation for quantum nutrition by showing that food, water, and cells interact through light.

Research on Food Quality and Biophoton Emissions

Studies confirm that the photonic quality of food matters as much as its biochemical profile:

- Fresh fruits and vegetables emit higher levels of biophotons than processed or irradiated foods [3].

- Sprouts and young plants exhibit the highest photon emission per gram, correlating with vitality and nutrient density [8].
- Post-harvest biophoton decay parallels nutrient loss, linking freshness with photon coherence [9].
- Weak luminescence studies show a strong relationship between food quality and ultraweak light emissions [3].

Implication: Measuring food photons could become a new nutritional biomarker beyond vitamins or calories.

Photobiomodulation and Cellular Nutrition

Light does not just radiate; it nourishes. Research in photobiomodulation (PBM) demonstrates that:

- Red/NIR light (600–950 nm) stimulates cytochrome c oxidase, enhancing mitochondrial ATP production [4].
- PBM reduces oxidative stress, improves tissue repair, and promotes neuroprotection [10].
- In animals and humans, PBM improves muscle recovery, cognition, and emotional balance [11,12].

These findings suggest that biophotons are functional nutrients capable of modulating metabolism, recovery, and resilience.

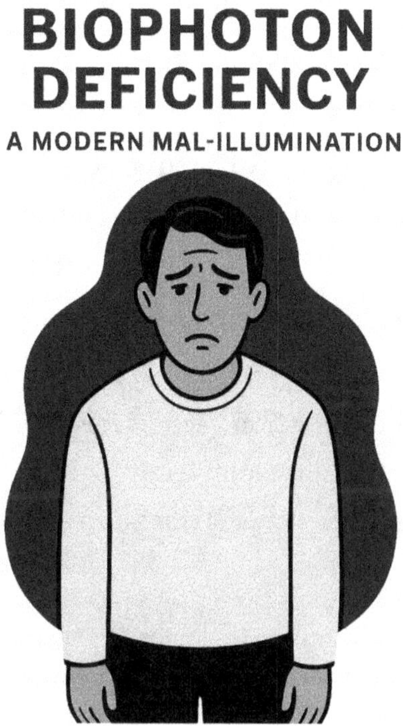

Figure 7.1. Biophoton Deficiency and Its Link to Chronic Disorders. *The illustration depicts a person with diminished radiance and low vitality, symbolizing biophoton deficiency, also referred to as "modern mal-illumination." A lack of coherent light within cells disrupts mitochondrial function, weakens the biofield, and contributes to fatigue, inflammation, and susceptibility to chronic disorders. This visual underscores the importance of restoring biophoton coherence as a foundation for health and disease prevention.*

Biophoton Deficiency and Chronic Disorders

Emerging evidence links low photon coherence to disease:

- Patients with cancer show chaotic or diminished photon emissions compared to healthy controls [1].
- Neurodegenerative diseases (e.g., Alzheimer's, Parkinson's) correlate with mitochondrial dysfunction and reduced photon output [13].

- Chronic fatigue and fibromyalgia patients show altered photon signatures, suggesting impaired energy metabolism [14].

Hypothesis: Many disorders may be reframed as "biophoton deficiency syndromes," where restoring photon flow could promote healing.

Current Research Directions in Quantum Nutrition

1. Food Biophysics
    - Photon emission analysis for quality grading and supply chain monitoring.
    - Structured water studies in fruits and vegetables.
2. Clinical Trials
    - Use of biophoton devices in chronic pain, neurodegeneration, diabetes, and fatigue.
    - Correlating food photon intake with HRV, mitochondrial function, and biofield scans.
3. Agricultural Applications
    - Photonic cultivation strategies for enhanced yields and nutrient density [15].
    - Reduced reliance on fertilizers and pesticides.
4. Biofield Imaging and Diagnostics
    - Gas Discharge Visualization (GDV), Kirlian photography, and CCD photon imaging to measure systemic coherence [5].
5. AI and Frequency Mapping
    - Integrating AI-driven biofield analytics with nutritional recommendations (see Chapter 19).

Case Example: Biophotons in Fresh vs. Processed Foods

In one controlled study, spinach leaves were tested immediately after harvest vs. after refrigeration. Photon emission dropped sharply after several days in cold storage, mirroring loss of chlorophyll and antioxidant activity [9].
Lesson: Food quality is not only chemical; it is quantum temporal coherence.

Summary: Research Validates Light as Nutrition

Research Focus	Key Finding	Relevance to Nutrition
Biophoton emission	Cells and foods emit coherent light [1,2,3]	Photon coherence is a biomarker of vitality
Food studies	Fresh/raw foods emit more photons [3,8]	High-photon foods enhance resilience
Photobiomodulation	Red/NIR light enhances ATP [4,10]	Light is a metabolic nutrient
Disease correlation	Low coherence in illness [1,13,14]	Chronic disease = photon deficiency
Agriculture	Photonic farming enhances yield [15]	Sustainable, high-quality crops

Quantum nutrition research confirms: To eat light is to restore coherence.

References

1. Popp FA. Biophoton emission: experimental background and theoretical approaches. *Modern Physics Letters B.* 1994;8(21-22):1269-1296.

2. van Wijk R, van Wijk EPA. Biophoton communication and regulation in living systems. *J Photochem Photobiol B.* 2005;79(2):141–147.

3. Quickenden TI, Hee SSQ. Weak luminescence from the yeast Saccharomyces cerevisiae and the existence of mitogenetic radiation. *Biochem Biophys Res Commun.*1974 Sep 23;60(2):764–70.

4. Hamblin MR. Mechanisms of photobiomodulation in human cells. *J Biophotonics.* 2017;10(11):1462–1481.

5. Rubik B. The biofield hypothesis: its biophysical basis and role in medicine. *J Altern Complement Med.* 2002;8(6):703–717.

6. Gurwitsch AG. Die Natur des spezifischen Erregers der Zellteilung. *Archiv für Entwicklungsmechanik der Organismen.* 1923;100:11-40. German.

7. Pollack GH. *The fourth phase of water.* Ebner & Sons; 2013.

8. Yan Y, Popp FA, Rothe GM. Correlation between germination capacity and biophoton emission of barley seeds (*Hordeum vulgare* L.). *Seed Science and Technology.* 2003;31(2):249-258.

9. Yamauchi N, Watada AE. Chlorophyll and xanthophyll changes in broccoli florets under storage. *Postharvest Biol Technol.* 1991;1(2):109–116.

10. Chung H, et al. The nuts and bolts of low-level laser therapy. *Ann Biomed Eng.* 2012;40(2):516–533.

11. Salehpour F, Cassano P. Transcranial photobiomodulation for cognition. *Neurophotonics.* 2021;8(2):022001.

12. Henderson TA, Morries LD. Near-infrared phototherapy for brain disorders. *Neuropsychiatr Dis Treat.* 2015;11:2191–2208.

13. Swerdlow RH. Mitochondria and neurodegeneration. *Science.* 2018;360(6386): 638–642.

14. Van Wijk EPA, et al. Biophoton emission in chronic fatigue syndrome patients. *Forsch Komplementmed.* 2010;17(1):17–23.

15. Kavipriya S, Beaulah A, Sundharaiya K, Anitha T, Sivakumar KP. The role of LED lighting in enhancing post-harvest fruit and vegetable quality. *Plant Science Today (Early Access).* May 2025. doi:10.14719/pst.7318

CHAPTER 8

Biophotons and Consciousness

Consciousness may arise not merely from the firing of neurons, but from the light that synchronizes them—biophotons weaving thought, perception, and awareness into a unified field of experience.

—James Z. Liu, MD, PhD

Introduction

Consciousness—the capacity to perceive, integrate, and respond to internal and external realities—remains one of the most profound mysteries of science. While neurobiology has provided detailed insights into the electrochemical mechanisms of neuronal signaling, a deeper layer of organization may exist at the quantum–biophysical level. Emerging evidence suggests that biophotons, ultra-weak photon emissions from living cells, may play a critical role in orchestrating consciousness by enabling coherent communication within and across neural networks.

This chapter explores the role of biophotons in consciousness, reviewing the evidence for their generation, pathways of transmission, influence on brain dynamics, and their possible relationship to subjective experience.

Biophotons in the Brain

Biophoton emissions, first discovered in plants and later verified in animal and human cells, have been measured in the brain, particularly in neuronal tissues rich in mitochondria and chromophores such as cytochrome oxidase and flavoproteins [1–3]. Studies using photomultiplier tubes and ultra-sensitive imaging systems show that neurons emit photons in the visible and near-infrared range (350–1,300 nm), often correlated with oxidative metabolic activity [4].

Importantly, the intensity of biophoton emissions in neural tissue is not random but exhibits patterned coherence, suggesting a potential role in neural signaling beyond conventional electrochemical synapses [5].

Axonal Transmission of Biophotons

Recent theoretical and experimental work has proposed that axons and myelinated nerve fibers may function as optical waveguides for biophotons [6–8]. The refractive index difference between axoplasm and the surrounding myelin sheath provides suitable conditions for guiding photons over long distances with minimal loss, akin to optical fibers in telecommunications.

It opens the possibility that the brain harbors a dual signaling system:

- Electrical: mediated by action potentials and neurotransmitters.
- Photonic: mediated by ultra-weak coherent photons traveling through axonal pathways.

Such a system could provide a substrate for high-speed, parallel information processing that transcends the limits of chemical synaptic transmission.

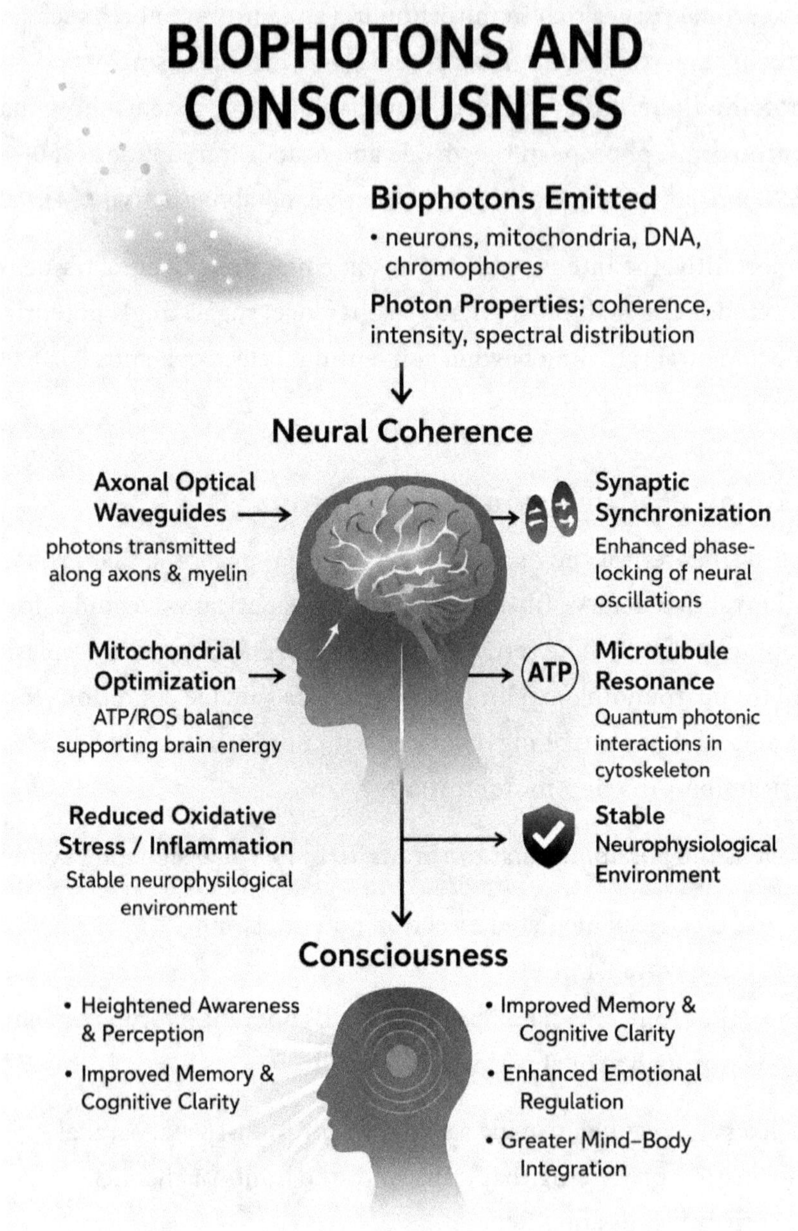

Figure 8.1. Biophotons and Consciousness. *Schematic representation of how biophoton emissions interact with neural substrates to generate coherence, synchronize brain networks, optimize mitochondrial and microtubule dynamics, and ultimately support conscious experience.*

Biophoton Coherence and Neural Synchronization

One hallmark of consciousness is synchronized oscillatory activity across distributed brain regions, particularly in gamma-band frequencies (30–100 Hz). Biophotons, by virtue of their coherence, may act as a physical medium for phase-locking neural assemblies [9].

Fritz-Albert Popp proposed that coherent photon fields could serve as a "biological laser," synchronizing cellular processes and perhaps even the collective firing of neuronal ensembles [10]. Experimental evidence supports this view, showing that stress, pathology, and aging are associated with a breakdown in coherence, while healthy tissue maintains orderly photon emissions [11].

Quantum Brain Models and Biophotons

Theories of consciousness, such as the Orchestrated Objective Reduction (Orch-OR) model by Hameroff and Penrose, emphasize quantum-level processes in microtubules as central to conscious awareness [12]. Biophotons may provide the missing bridge, interacting with microtubules to sustain coherence and facilitate quantum information transfer [13].

Microtubules are known to absorb and emit photons, and their ordered lattice structure may allow for photonic entanglement and resonance effects [14]. In this framework, biophotons act not only as carriers of energy but also as carriers of information, potentially linked to the emergence of conscious states.

Consciousness, Biofields, and Biophotons

Beyond neural signaling, biophotons may contribute to a biofield, a subtle electromagnetic and photonic field proposed to underlie systemic regulation and mind–body interactions [15]. Some experimental studies have shown correlations between meditation, altered states of consciousness, and changes in ultra-weak photon emissions [16]. These findings suggest that subjective states of consciousness may modulate biophoton activity, and conversely, coherent photonic signaling may stabilize conscious awareness.

Clinical and Therapeutic Implications

If biophotons are indeed central to consciousness, therapeutic interventions aimed at restoring photonic coherence may help treat disorders of consciousness, such as:

- Neurodegenerative diseases (Alzheimer's, Parkinson's) [17–22]
- Post-stroke cognitive impairment [23–25]
- Traumatic brain injury (TBI) [26,27]
- Mood disorders linked to dysregulated brain networks.

Preliminary studies using biophoton generators and low-level photonic therapies report improvements in cognition, attention, physiological activities, and emotional regulation [17–29]. These early findings underscore the potential of Biophoton Quantum Medicine to open new frontiers in consciousness research and clinical care.

Conclusion

Biophotons provide a compelling framework for linking the material brain to the immaterial mind. Acting as coherent information carriers, they may synchronize neural networks, interact with quantum structures such as microtubules, and contribute to the biofield underlying systemic consciousness. While the evidence remains preliminary, biophoton research offers a promising path toward unraveling one of humanity's greatest mysteries: the origin and mechanisms of consciousness.

References

1. Kobayashi M. et. al. Imaging of ultraweak spontaneous photon emission from human body displaying diurnal rhythm. *PLoS ONE.* 2009;4(7):e6256. doi:10.1371/journal.pone.0006256, 2009.

2. Isojima Y, Isoshima T, Nagai K, Kikuchi K, Nakagawa H. Ultraweak biochemiluminescence detected from rat hippocampal slices. *Neuroreport.* 1995;6(4):658–660.

3. van Wijk R, van Wijk EPA, Wiegant FAC, Ives J. Free radicals and low-level photon emission in human pathophysiology: new concepts in diagnosis and therapy. *J Altern Complement Med.* 2008;14(4):333-338.

4. Tang R, Dai J. Spatiotemporal imaging of glutamate-induced biophotonic activities and transmission in neural circuits. *PLoS One.* 2014;9(1):e85643.

5. Wang C, Bókkon I, Dai J, Antal I. Spontaneous ultra-weak photon emission and delayed luminescence of human brain. *J Photochem Photobiol B.* 2016;159:109–116.

6. Kumar S, Boone K, Tuszyński JA, Barclay P, Simon C. Possible existence of optical communication channels in the brain. *Sci Rep.* 2016;6:36508.

7. Bókkon I, Salari V, Tuszyński J, Antal I. Estimation of the number of biophotons involved in the visual perception of a single-object image. *J Photochem Photobiol B.* 2010;100(1):1–8.

8. Rahnama M, Tuszyński J, Bókkon I, Cifra M, Sardar P, Salari V. Emission of mitochondrial biophotons and neural activity of the brain. *Neural Regen Res.* 2011;6(6):430–439.

9. Jibu M, Hagan S, Hameroff SR, Pribram KH, Yasue K. Quantum optical coherence in cytoskeletal microtubules: implications for brain function. *Biosystems.* 1994;32(3):195–209.

10. Popp FA. About the coherence of biophotons. *Radiat Environ Biophys.* 1979;16(3):199–210.

11. van Wijk EPA, van Wijk R. Multi-site recording and spectral analysis of spontaneous photon emission from human body. *Forsch Komplementmed.* 2005;12(2):96–106.

12. Hameroff S, Penrose R. Consciousness in the universe: A review of the 'Orch OR' theory. *Phys Life Rev.* 2014;11(1):39–78.

13. Bókkon I, Salari V, Tuszyński J, Antal I. Estimation of the number of biophotons involved in the visual perception of a single-object image: biophoton intensity can be considerably higher inside cells than outside. *J Photochem Photobiol B.* 2010 Sep 2;100(3):160–6.

14. Jibu M, Yasue K. What is mind? Quantum field theory of evanescent photons in brain as quantum theory of consciousness. *Informatica.* 1995;19(3):471–490.

15. Rubik B. The biofield hypothesis: Its biophysical basis and role in medicine. *J Altern Complement Med.* 2002;8(6):703–717.

16. Van Wijk EPA, Van Wijk R, Bosman S, Van der Greef J. Human ultra-weak photon emission and the level of consciousness. *Conscious Cogn.* 2008;17(4):1223–1233.

17. Liu JZ, Smotrys MA, Robinson SD, Yu HX, Sherry X Liu SX, Liu DR, and Gu HY. Multimodal evidence of cognitive

restoration in Alzheimer's disease following biophoton therapy: A neurophysiological and energetic assessment. Multimodal. *J Alzheimers Dise & Rep.* 2025;2(3):1–10.

18. Liu JZ, Smotrys MA, Robinson SD, Yu HX, Sherry X Liu SX, Liu DR, and Gu HY. Quantitative EEG evidence of cognitive restoration in Alzheimer's disease following biophoton generator therapy. *J Neurol Res Rev Rep.* 2025;7(7):1–7.

19. Hu Y., Chien L, Gu HY, and Liu JZ. Enhancing blood fluidity and physiological markers in early-stage Alzheimer's disease using biophoton generators: A case study. *Journal of Neurology Research Reviews & Reports.* 2025, 7(7): 1-7.

20. Liu JZ, Smotrys M, Robinson SD, Liu S, Gu HY. Therapeutic benefits of biophoton therapy in Parkinson's disease: Clinical evidence from a pilot and real-world study. *J Neurol Res Rev Rep.* 2025;7(6):1–6.

21. Liu JZ, Smotrys MA, Robinson SD, Yu HX, Sherry X Liu SX, Liu DR, and Gu HY. Quantitative EEG evidence of functional brain recovery in Parkinson's disease following biophoton therapy. *J Neurol Res Rev Rep.* 2025;7(7):14–20.

22. Hu Y, Gu HY, Liu JZ. Twelve-day live blood analysis reveals hemorheological and microvascular restoration in a Parkinson's disease patient following biophoton therapy. *Journal of Neurology Research Reviews & Reports.* 2025;(7):219.

23. Liu JZ, Smotrys MA, Robinson SD, Yu HX, Sherry X Liu SX, Liu DR, and Gu HY. A breakthrough in stroke rehabilitation: Non-invasive biophoton therapy promotes neurofunctional recovery in chronic stroke patients. *J Alzheimers Dise & Rep 2025, 2(3): 1-3.*

24. Liu JZ, Smotrys MA, Robinson SD, Yu HX, Sherry X Liu SX, Liu DR, and Gu HY. Quantitative EEG reveals cognitive and motor restoration after biophoton treatment in chronic stroke. *J Neurol Res Rev Rep.* 2025;7(8):1–10.

25. Hu Y., Chien L, Gu HY, and Liu JZ. Enhancing blood fluidity and physiological markers in chronic stroke using biophoton generators: A case study. *Journal of Neurology Research Reviews & Reports. SRC/JNRRR*. 2025;281. doi:10.47363/JNRRR/2025(7)223

26. Hu Y, Chien L, Gu HY, Liu JZ (2025). Biophoton therapy restores hemorheology in chronic stroke: Live blood evidence of microvascular recovery. *Journal of Neurology Research Reviews & Reports. SRC/JNRRR*. 2025;287. doi:10.47363/JNRRR/2025(7)229

27. Liu JZ, Smotrys MA, Robinson SD, Yu HX, Sherry X Liu SX, Liu DR, and Gu HY. Biophoton therapy reverses electrophysiological deficits in chronic traumatic brain injury: Quantitative EEG evidence of cognitive and network recovery. *J Neurol Res Rev Rep.* 2025;7(8):1–11.

28. Thomas T, Gu HY, Smotrys MA, Robinson SD, and Liu JZ. Non-Invasive biophoton therapy for neurocognitive and physical recovery in retired athletes with traumatic brain injury: A pilot study in former NFL players. *Journal of Neurology Research Reviews & Reports. SRC/JNRRR*. 2025;288.

29. Liu JZ, Gu HY, Hu Y, Smotrys M, Robinson SD. Safety and efficacy of biophoton quantum medicine in treating neurodegenerative diseases. *J Neurol Res Rev Rep.* 2025;7(7):1–6.

30. Liu JZ, Gu HY, Smotrys M and Robinson SD. Harnessing biophoton energy: A novel paradigm to treat unmet medical conditions. *Mod Appro Drug Des.* 2025;4(4). MADD. 000595

CHAPTER 9

Biophotons and Frequencies in Nourishment

Beyond Calories: The Photonic Architecture of True Biological Nourishment

---

Nourishment is not merely the transfer of molecules; it is the transfer of biological information carried through light.

—James Z. Liu, MD, PhD

Introduction

Nutrition has historically been defined in terms of macronutrients (carbohydrates, proteins, and fats) and micronutrients (vitamins and minerals). However, growing evidence suggests that light itself—carried as biophotons and structured electromagnetic frequencies—constitutes an essential and previously overlooked dimension of nourishment. Foods, beverages, and natural environments are not merely chemical substrates but also carriers of photonic and vibrational information that modulate biological function. This chapter explores the concept of biophotons and frequencies in nourishment, their scientific basis, and their implications for health and longevity.

Biophotons in Living Systems

Biophotons are ultra-weak light emissions in the visible and ultraviolet ranges, produced by living cells as by-products of metabolic and oxidative processes. First described as "mitogenetic radiation" by Gurwitsch in 1923 and later elaborated on by Fritz-Albert Popp in the 1970s, biophotons have since been confirmed as coherent, low-level emissions that regulate cellular communication, DNA function, and physiological homeostasis.

- Fresh fruits, vegetables, and raw foods exhibit stronger biophoton emissions compared to processed foods, correlating with vitality and nutrient density.
- Biophoton coherence, rather than intensity alone, appears to determine biological efficacy, reflecting ordered molecular structures within the food matrix.

Thus, the quality of nourishment is not only chemical but photonic, with biophotons acting as carriers of information that sustain life processes beyond caloric energy.

Frequencies and Nutritional Resonance

Beyond biophotons, biological systems respond to a range of electromagnetic frequencies. Resonant frequencies can modulate enzymatic activity, mitochondrial function, and even gene expression.

- Structured water within cells acts as a liquid crystalline matrix, responsive to light frequencies, storing and transmitting vibrational information.
- The cytoskeleton and membranes exhibit vibrational coherence that enables long-range communication across tissues.
- Nutritional inputs, when exposed to sunlight or coherent light, can enhance photonic qualities and bioavailability.

This view reframes nourishment as frequency exchange, where food and light interact dynamically to optimize metabolic efficiency and coherence.

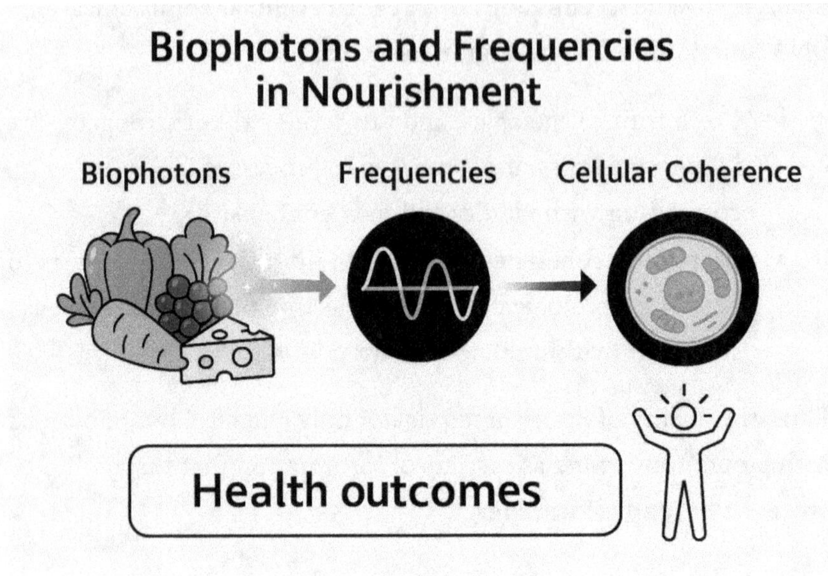

Figure 9.1. Biophotons and Frequencies in Nourishment. *This schematic illustrates how food acts as more than just a source of molecular nutrients but also carries biophotons—ultra-weak photons emitted by living systems—that deliver frequencies essential for regulating cellular coherence. Biophotons absorbed from nutrient-rich, fresh foods interact with cellular systems to optimize mitochondrial energy production, enhance intercellular communication, and restore systemic order. Through this photonic information transfer, frequencies guide biological processes, sustaining coherence across tissues and supporting optimal health outcomes such as resilience, vitality, and disease resistance. This model underscores the dual role of nourishment, molecular and photonic, in maintaining human health.*

Biophotons and Mitochondrial Nourishment

Mitochondria are key absorbers of light, especially through cytochrome c oxidase (CCO), which is sensitive to red and near-infrared wavelengths. This interaction improves ATP production, reduces oxidative stress, and modulates signaling pathways. Thus, foods rich in biophotons and environments rich in sunlight may synergize to support mitochondrial bioenergetics, the fundamental engine of cellular vitality.

Practical Implications: Food as Light Nutrition

1. Freshness matters: The fresher the food, the higher the biophoton emission, reflecting nutritional vitality.
2. Processing reduces coherence: Cooking, irradiation, and long-term storage diminish biophotonic content.
3. Sunlight as a nutrient: Direct exposure to natural light entrains circadian rhythms, stimulates vitamin D synthesis, and enhances endogenous biophoton production.
4. Synergy of diet and light: A diet rich in raw, fresh, and minimally processed foods, combined with daily natural light exposure, creates a photonic foundation for resilience.

Future Directions

The emerging field of Biophoton Quantum Nutrition seeks to integrate biophoton science, quantum biology, and nutrition. Potential areas of research include:

- Biophoton-based food quality testing, using ultra-sensitive detectors to evaluate vitality.
- Photonic supplementation, via biophoton generators or coherent light exposure, to enhance nutritional assimilation.
- Frequency-based dietary personalization, tailoring foods and light exposure to optimize biofield coherence and prevent disease.

Conclusion

Biophotons and frequencies represent a missing dimension of nourishment, bridging the gap between molecular nutrition and quantum biology. Recognizing light as a nutrient expands our understanding of food quality, metabolic health, and holistic well-being. Just as vitamins were once an overlooked aspect of nutrition, biophotons and frequency resonance may soon be recognized as essential for human vitality and longevity.

References

1. Gurwitsch, A. *Die mitogenetische strahlung*. Berlin: Springer; 1923.

2. Popp, F. A., Nagl, W., Li, K. H., Scholz, W., Weingärtner, O., & Wolf, R. Biophoton emission: New evidence for coherence and DNA as source. *Cell Biophysics.* 1984;6(1):33–52.

3. Popp, F. A., & Beloussov, L. V. (Eds.). *Integrative biophysics: Biophotonics.* Springer; 2003.

4. van Wijk, R. *Light in shaping life: Biophotons in biology and medicine.* Meluna Research; 2014.

5. Hamblin, M. R. Shining light on the head: Photobiomodulation for brain disorders. *BBA Clinical.* 2016;6:113–124.

6. Albrecht-Buehler, G. Cellular infrared detector appears to be contained in the centrosome. *Cell Motility and the Cytoskeleton,* 1994;27(3): 262–271.

7. Ho, M. W. *The rainbow and the worm: The physics of organisms.* World Scientific; 1998.

8. Pollack, G. H. *The fourth phase of water: Beyond solid, liquid, and vapor.* Ebner and Sons; 2013.

9. Scholkmann, F., Fels, D., & Cifra, M. Non-chemical and non-contact cell-to-cell communication: A short review. *American Journal of Translational Research,* 2013;5(6):586–593.

PART II

The Quantum Nature of Nutrients

Part II explores how food and environment act not only as sources of matter but as carriers of light, frequency, and biological information—what we now recognize as *quantum nutrients.* These chapters reveal how nourishment extends beyond chemistry into the realm of biophotonics, resonance, and structured coherence.

Chapter 10 reframes *food as information,* emphasizing how nutrients carry encoded signals that guide DNA expression, cellular repair, and systemic regulation.

Chapter 11 examines the *photon profile of living foods,* showing how fresh, unprocessed, and sun-ripened plants emit coherent light that directly enhances biological vitality.

Chapter 12 investigates *water as a quantum medium,* revealing how structured water stores and transmits photonic energy, essential for hydration, enzymatic activity, and cellular communication.

Chapter 13 highlights *sunlight as a master nutrient,* not only fueling photosynthesis but regulating circadian rhythms, hormone production, and mitochondrial performance.

Chapter 14 introduces protocols for *combining biophoton exposures*—through food, light therapies, and structured environments—to amplify healing effects and restore systemic coherence.

Chapter 15 details methods for *measuring progress,* including biological age reversal, energy field imaging, and coherence-based biomarkers that reflect quantum nutritional outcomes.

Chapter 16 expands the horizon into *biophotonic medicine,* discussing how this emerging science may reshape aging research, longevity clinics, AI-assisted diagnostics, and even global wellness systems.

Chapter 17 addresses *deglycation and detoxification* through quantum inputs, showing how coherent energy helps reverse molecular damage, reduce oxidative burden, and restore cellular resilience.

Together, these chapters establish a revolutionary perspective: nutrients are not only matter but messages, not only calories but coherence. By integrating food, water, light, and frequency into a unified framework, Part II shows how quantum nutrition can unlock the body's regenerative capacity, slow aging, and build a foundation for global health innovation.

CHAPTER 10

Food as Information

Beyond Calories—Understanding the Quantum Code of Nourishment

---

Don't count the calories. Count the coherence.

—James Z. Liu, MD, PhD

What If Your Body Reads Food?

In classical nutrition, food is reduced to measurable components: carbohydrates, fats, proteins, vitamins, and minerals. The paradigm is numeric: *calories in, calories out.* But from a quantum perspective, food is far more than fuel; it is information, encoded in light, structure, vibration, and frequency [1,2].

Your body is not a passive chemical factory. It is an intelligent, self-regulating field that interprets its environment. Every meal delivers encoded biological messages, and your cells listen, decode, and respond. Food choices, therefore, are not just about macronutrients but about which *instructions* you choose to transmit to your body.

The Quantum Information in Food

Every whole food—plant, seed, fruit, or animal product—carries more than atoms. It contains:

- Biophoton emissions: light-encoded information from metabolic processes [3,4].

- Molecular vibrations: electromagnetic oscillations from chemical bonds [5].
- Fractal geometries and sacred ratios: e.g., Fibonacci spirals in sunflower seeds and broccoli florets, reflecting self-organizing principles in nature [6].
- Epigenetic signals: bioactive compounds that influence gene expression [7].
- Quantum entanglement with environment: food carries imprints of its soil, sun, and ecosystem [2].

This informational matrix forms the food's quantum signature. When consumed intact, it provides not only nutrients but also a coherent data stream that supports stem cell activation, hormone regulation, and immune balance.

Why Processed Food Is Energetically "Empty"

A processed snack may still contain protein, fiber, or synthetic vitamins, but its informational integrity is often degraded. When food is:

- Microwaved
- Chemically treated
- Genetically modified
- Irradiated
- Mass-produced under artificial lighting

...it loses quantum coherence. Biophoton emissions drop, vibrational signatures flatten, and structural geometry collapses [3,4]. The result: food that feeds the body's *mass* but starves its *field.*

This explains why people can overeat processed foods yet remain energetically malnourished, fatigued, inflamed, and emotionally flat. Their systems crave not just calories but information.

Food as an Instruction Manual

Every bite of food transmits instructions to your cells. Nutrigenomics already confirms that food compounds regulate gene expression [7,8]. Quantum nutrition expands this idea: these instructions are not only chemical but also bioelectromagnetic.

Examples:

- Broccoli sprouts: sulforaphane activates Nrf2, a detoxification and cellular defense pathway.
- Blueberries: antioxidants modulate brain wave activity, enhancing memory and mood [9].
- Turmeric: curcumin regulates over 100 genes involved in inflammation and repair.
- Raw honey: encodes vibrational signatures from plants, bees, and sunlight [10].

Each food carries a unique frequency profile that either supports or disrupts the body's internal coherence.

The Power of Living Structure

In quantum biology, structure = information. The arrangement of atoms determines vibration, resonance, and signal quality.

Living-structured foods include:

- Raw vegetables with intact cell walls.
- Fresh fruits with natural symmetry.
- Fermented foods with microbial ecosystems.
- Sprouts and microgreens undergoing active division.

These foods preserve fractal and geometric intelligence, delivering rich informational input. In contrast, ultra-processed foods are structurally degraded and largely "silent" to the body's information systems.

Resonance Between Food and the Body

Each organ system vibrates at characteristic frequencies. When food's informational profile matches these frequencies, coherence is enhanced.

Food Type	Primary Frequency Resonance	Organ System Influenced
Leafy greens	528 Hz (DNA repair)	Heart and circulation
Berries, grapes	432 Hz (natural harmonic)	Brain and nervous system
Sea vegetables	7.83 Hz (Earth's Schumann resonance)	Thyroid and endocrine
Ginger, turmeric	Infrared (~9–12 μm)	Digestion and immunity

Selecting foods by resonance allows for precision nourishment, fine-tuning systems without drugs.

How to Choose Information-Rich Foods

To maximize food's informational value, follow the Five Quantum Guidelines:

1. Fresh is best: Eat within 48 hours of harvest; photon count drops quickly [4].
2. Honor natural structure: Choose whole, geometrically intact foods.
3. Eat the rainbow: Colors correspond to frequency bands; a varied spectrum nourishes widely.

4. Source locally: Local foods carry environmental signatures that train your immune field.
5. Program with intention: Bless, pray, or give thanks—consciousness imprints vibrational order [11].

Case Example: Rebuilding Vitality with Information-First Eating

A 48-year-old man recovering from long COVID reported brain fog and exhaustion despite a high-protein, low-carb diet and supplements. Lab tests were normal.

By shifting to an information-rich diet, including:

- Daily microgreens and sprouts,
- Sun-charged herbal infusions,
- Fresh-pressed juices consumed immediately,
- Eliminating microwaved meals,
- Short biophoton-generator sessions each morning,

He experienced within two weeks:

- Sharper focus,
- Increased energy,
- Reduced inflammation markers,
- Improved HRV and sleep cycles.

His recovery came not from calorie shifts but from clearer informational input.

Summary: Eat the Signal, Not Just the Substance

Quantum nutrition reframes food as a messenger system:

- It speaks in light, vibration, and geometry.

- It encodes instructions that guide healing and coherence.
- Its value is lost when reduced to numbers or denatured by processing.

You are not only what you eat; you are what your cells understand from what you eat.

The next chapter explores the photon profile of different foods, showing why some radiate vitality while others drain energy. It also introduces the Biophoton Emission Index as a tool for selecting the most life-enhancing foods.

References

1. Popp FA, Beloussov LV. *Integrative biophysics: Biophotonics.* Springer; 2003.
2. van Wijk R. *Light in shaping life: Biophotons in biology and medicine.* Meluna; 2014.
3. Cifra M, Pospíšil P. Ultra-weak photon emission from biological samples. *J Photochem Photobiol B.* 2014;139:2–10.
4. Scholkmann F, et al. Ultraweak photon emission as a non-invasive health assessment method. *J Photochem Photobiol B.* 2013;139:2–10.
5. Bajpai RP. Quantum coherence of biophotons and living systems. *Indian J Exp Biol.* 2003;41(5):514–527.
6. Thompson D. *On growth and form.* Cambridge Univ Press; 1942.
7. Kaput J, Rodriguez RL. Nutritional genomics: The next frontier in the postgenomic era. *Physiol Genomics.* 2004;16:166–177.

8. Ferguson LR. Nutrigenomics approaches to functional foods. *J Am Diet Assoc.* 2009;109(3):452–458.

9. Lopresti AL, Smith SJ, Pouchieu C, Pourtau L, Gaudout D, Pallet V, Drummond PD. Effects of a polyphenol-rich grape and blueberry extract (MemophenolTM) on cognitive function in older adults with mild cognitive impairment: A randomized, double-blind, placebo-controlled study. *Front Psychol.* 2023;14:1144231.

10. Al-Waili N, et al. Effects of natural honey on metabolic and cardiovascular risk factors. *J Med Food.* 2013;16(7):587–594.

11. Emoto M. *The hidden messages in water.* Beyond Words; 2004.

CHAPTER 11

The Photon Profile of Living Foods

Why Some Foods Radiate Life—And Others Drain It

Vital food is radiant food. If it doesn't shine, it can't nourish the light within you.
—James Z. Liu, MD, PhD

Why Some Foods Energize and Others Deplete

We've seen that food carries quantum information: biophotons, molecular vibrations, and electromagnetic signatures. But why do some meals leave you feeling clear and vibrant, while others make you sluggish, even if the nutrient breakdown looks "perfect"?

The answer lies in a food's photon profile, its unique light-emission signature that reflects its coherence, vitality, and bioenergetic compatibility [1,2]. The higher and more ordered a food's photon emission, the more it strengthens your biofield, improves cellular communication, and restores natural energy flow.

In quantum nutrition, food choice is not just about grams and calories. It is about light quality.

What Is a Photon Profile?

A photon profile refers to the intensity, coherence, and spectral distribution of ultraweak photon emissions (biophotons) from living food. These emissions:

- Occur in the UV to visible spectrum (200–1200 nm).
- Are continuous in all biological systems.
- Reflect the food's energetic order and informational integrity [1,3].

High-photon foods share common traits:

- Grown in natural sunlight.
- Freshly harvested and intact.
- Not cooked, irradiated, or genetically modified.
- Rich in structured water and coherent cellular membranes.

By contrast, low-photon foods may still provide chemical nutrients but lack energetic intelligence, offering little resonance to the human system.

The Science Behind Food-Light Emissions

German biophysicist Fritz-Albert Popp pioneered the study of food biophotons. His findings included:

- Organic, fresh produce emits significantly more coherent light than conventionally farmed or processed food [2].
- Biophoton intensity declines rapidly after harvest, especially under refrigeration or mechanical cutting.
- Foods with strong coherence support DNA repair, mitochondrial efficiency, and immune communication [4].

Popp concluded that biophotons act as a regulatory network and that foods rich in coherent light help restore biological order.

The Biophoton Emission Index (BEI)

To translate this science into practice, we introduce the Biophoton Emission Index (BEI), a relative ranking system of foods by their light emission profile:

BEI Rank	Food Type	Photon Profile
🌟🌟🌟🌟🌟 (Highest)	Fresh sprouts, raw greens, wild herbs, sun-ripened berries	Highly coherent, photon-rich, life-enhancing
🌟🌟🌟🌟	Raw fruits, fresh-pressed juices, fermented vegetables	Strong emissions, support microbiome and repair
🌟🌟🌟	Lightly cooked organic vegetables, soaked seeds	Moderate photon retention, structurally intact
🌟🌟	Refrigerated produce, bottled juices	Photon-depleted, less vitality
🌟 (Lowest)	Microwaved meals, processed snacks, irradiated foods	Chaotic, incoherent emissions; biofield-draining

This ranking reframes "nutritional density" not only as chemical, but also as quantum vitality.

Foods That Radiate Life

Examples of naturally high-photon foods:

- Broccoli sprouts: among the highest photon emitters per gram.
- Sun-ripened tomatoes: store light energy in pigments and skin.
- Wild blueberries: fractal pigment distribution and dense antioxidants.

- Fermented sauerkraut: rhythmic photon pulses linked to microbial ecosystems [5].
- Fresh herbs: rosemary, basil, and cilantro show sharp, structured emission peaks.

These foods are alive when consumed, structurally intact, and deeply connected to sunlight, Earth resonance, and microbial activity.

What Dims a Food's Light?

1. Time After Harvest

- Biophoton levels decline steeply after picking.
- Spinach, for example, loses more than 50% of its coherence after 48 hours of refrigeration [2].

2. Cooking Method

- Steaming preserves more photon structure than boiling or frying.
- Microwaving disrupts vibrational order, producing chaotic emission patterns [6].

3. Processing

- Pasteurization, homogenization, and chemical additives degrade photon signals.
- Nutrients remain, but quantum information is lost.

4. Irradiation and Genetic Modification

- Irradiation sterilizes food by damaging DNA, collapsing photon patterns.
- Genetically modified foods often display irregular, incoherent emissions [7].

Enhancing the Photon Profile of Meals

You don't need a personal greenhouse to access high-photon foods daily. Simple practices help restore vitality:

- Sun-charging: Place fruits, herbs, or water in natural sunlight for 20–30 minutes.
- Structured hydration: Rinse is made with structured water to refresh its field.
- Eat seasonally and locally: Locally grown food resonates with your environmental field.
- Mindful preparation: Cook or prepare with calm, gratitude, and presence; intention itself influences crystalline structure [8].
- Avoid microwaves: Reheat gently with steam, on the stovetop, or in an infrared oven.

Even small upgrades in preparation yield large energetic returns.

Case Example: Chronic Bloating Reversed by High-Photon Eating

A 34-year-old woman experienced chronic bloating, fatigue, and dull skin. Tests showed mild dysbiosis, but her diet—protein shakes, packaged bars, and steamed vegetables—was chemically sound.

By shifting to a photon-first diet, including:

- Raw greens with sun-charged lemon water in the morning,
- Home-fermented sauerkraut and microgreens daily,
- Elimination of microwaved meals, and
- Sleeping with a biophoton generator,

...she reported improvements within 10 days: reduced bloating, elevated energy, glowing skin, and emotional uplift. She described feeling "plugged back in." The difference came from restoring field coherence, not changing macronutrients.

Summary: Choose Light, Choose Life

Quantum Principle	Nutritional Translation
Life is regulated by coherent light	Eat photon-rich, fresh foods.
Structure encodes information	Choose whole, geometric, unprocessed foods.
Photon emission = vitality	Prioritize raw, sun-grown, and fermented foods.
Cooking alters energy	Use gentle cooking to preserve vibrational order.
Your field eats too	Prepare and eat food with gratitude and awareness.

In quantum nutrition, food is not just sustenance; it is a photonic event. To heal, thrive, and renew vitality, we must eat not just for survival, but for light.

The next chapter will turn to water, often neglected in modern nutrition, and reveal how structured water acts as a quantum conductor, transforming hydration into a powerful carrier of light and information.

References

1. Popp FA, Beloussov LV. *Integrative biophysics: Biophotonics.* Springer; 2003.
2. van Wijk R. *Light in shaping life: Biophotons in biology and medicine.* Meluna; 2014.

3. Cifra M, Pospíšil P. Ultra-weak photon emission from biological samples: mechanisms and applications. *J Photochem Photobiol B*. 2014;139:2–10.

4. Scholkmann F, et al. Ultraweak photon emission as a diagnostic tool. *J Photochem Photobiol B*. 2013;139:2–10.

5. Fels D. Cellular communication through light: food and microbial studies. *PLoS One*. 2009;4(4):e5086.

6. Bajpai RP. Coherence of biophotons and the effects of microwaves. *Indian J Exp Biol*. 2003;41(5):514–527.

7. Popp FA. Biophoton emission as a measure of food quality. In: *Recent advances in biophoton research and its applications*. World Scientific; 1992.

8. Emoto M. *The hidden messages in water*. Beyond Words Publishing; 2004.

CHAPTER 12

Water, Structure, and Light

The Quantum Conductor of Life's Information

Water is not just a solvent—it's a living matrix, a light-encoded carrier of energy and consciousness.
—Dr. Gerald Pollack

Water: More Than Hydration

In conventional nutrition, water is often treated as background—essential for circulation, hydration, and temperature regulation. However, from a quantum perspective, water is not a passive substance. It is an active conductor of life, organizing energy, frequency, and information across the body [1].

Every biological function—digestion, immunity, energy metabolism—depends not only on *how much water* you drink, but also on the quality of that water: whether it is structured, coherent, and capable of transmitting light and bioinformation.

Water as a Living Matrix

By number of molecules, the human body is nearly 99% water [2]. For decades, water was regarded as a neutral solvent. Yet pioneering research, especially from Dr. Gerald Pollack's laboratory, shows that intracellular water is ordered, structured, and dynamically responsive to light [3].

This structured state, known as Exclusion Zone (EZ) water, forms next to hydrophilic surfaces such as membranes and proteins. EZ water:

- Arranges into hexagonal molecular lattices,
- Stores electrical charge,
- Excludes toxins and solutes, and
- Captures and transfers light and electromagnetic energy [3,4].

In this way, water behaves like a liquid crystal, aligning with and amplifying the body's coherent electromagnetic fields.

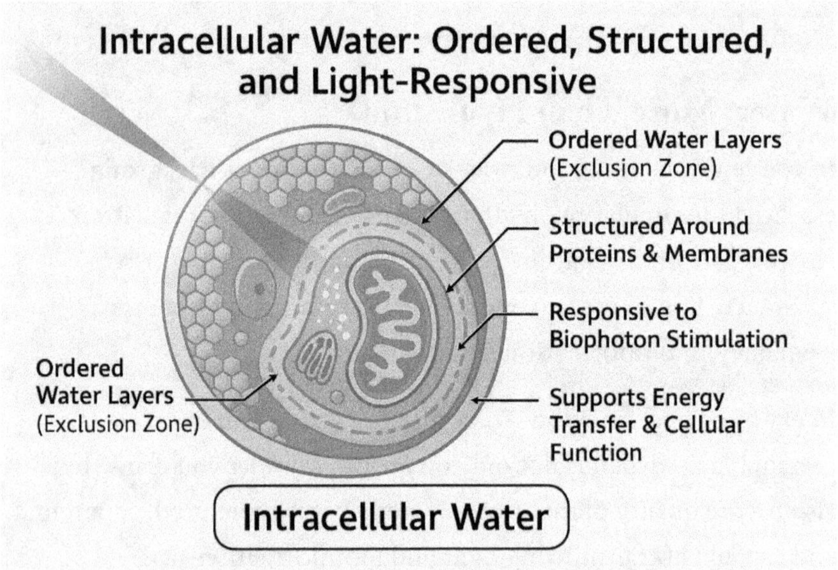

Figure 12.1. A Magnified Cell Cutaway Highlighting Intracellular Water. *Intracellular water is ordered, structured, and dynamically responsive to light. Biophoton stimulation enhances the organization of water layers around proteins, membranes, and mitochondria, supporting energy transfer and optimal cellular function.*

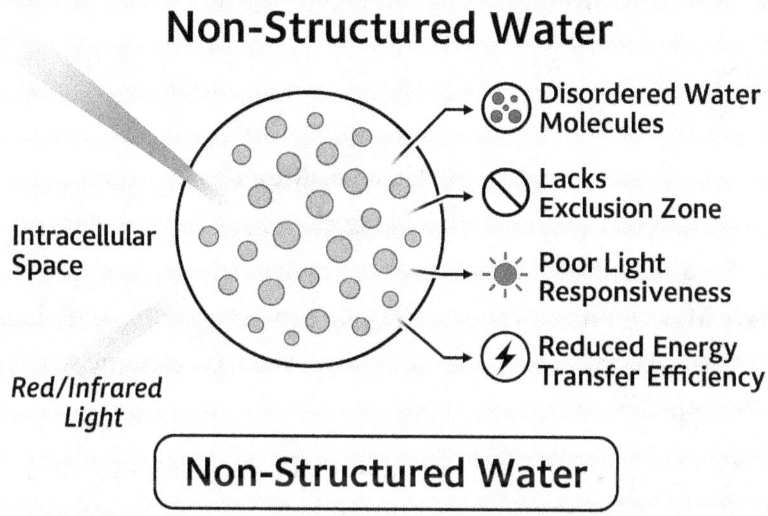

Figure 12.2. Non-Structured Water. *Non-structured intracellular water lacks ordered layers and coherence. Disordered water molecules exhibit poor responsiveness to light, weak exclusion zones, and reduced energy-transfer efficiency, which limits cellular function compared to structured water.*

Water as a Biophoton Carrier

Biophotons, the ultraweak light emitted by cells, require a medium for transmission. Water provides this medium.

- Structured water allows faster, more coherent photon transfer than disordered water [5].
- Water clusters can store photonic data, functioning like a biological memory chip.
- The vibrational state of water determines how it responds to food, thoughts, and environmental energy [6].

Water does not merely hydrate; it communicates.

Water's Memory and Transformation

The possibility that water stores information has long fascinated scientists.

- Jacques Benveniste and later Luc Montagnier (Nobel Laureate) suggested that water can retain electromagnetic signatures of substances, even when chemically absent [7].
- Masaru Emoto's crystallography experiments illustrated that words, emotions, and music alter water's crystalline structure [8].

Though controversial, these findings support the view that water is consciousness-sensitive and capable of storing subtle bioinformation.

In quantum nutrition, this means:

- Water carries messages from food, light, environment, and intention.
- The structure of water in your cells determines how efficiently those messages are received.

Signs of Quantum-Level Dehydration

Sometimes fatigue, inflammation, or brain fog persist even when water intake is high. This reflects not a lack of volume but a loss of water structure. Signs include:

- Persistent fatigue despite rest.
- Brain fog and memory lapses.
- Chronic inflammation or sluggish detox.
- Dull skin and brittle hair.

Here, the solution is not "more water." It is coherent water.

Sources of Structured, Coherent Water

Source	Benefits
Spring water (natural, unprocessed)	Mineral-rich, naturally charged, highly structured.
Vegetable water (cucumber, celery, aloe)	Bound to plant biofields; absorbed efficiently.
Glacial meltwater	Hexagonal geometry, energized by sunlight.
Biophoton-charged water	Structured by coherent light (e.g., sunlight, Tesla BioHealers).
Hydrogen-rich water	Antioxidant effects support mitochondrial hydration.
Vortexed or spun water	Mimics river motion, restores hexagonal structuring.

These forms of water are quantum-active, delivering both hydration and energy.

How to Structure Water at Home

Even without access to mountain springs, you can restore vitality to ordinary water:

1. Exposure to morning sunlight: place a glass of water in the sun for 30 minutes.
2. Use sound frequencies: play solfeggio tones or healing music near water.
3. Add natural elements: quartz, shungite, or mineral salts (with purity assurance).
4. Vortex stirring: Stir vigorously in a clockwise direction, then in a counterclockwise direction.
5. Infuse with intention: speak gratitude or offer a prayer; the water responds structurally [8].

These methods restore charge, coherence, and bioavailability, transforming water into quantum nutrition.

Water in Food: Hidden Quantum Nutrition

Many high-photon foods are also rich in structured water. Plants structure their own water through photosynthesis and biofield interaction.

- Cucumbers, watermelon, aloe vera, and coconut water contain gel-like water that hydrates more efficiently than plain liquid [9].
- Cooking denatures this water, reducing vibrational quality.

Eating raw, water-rich foods is a direct way to increase both hydration and biophotonic intake.

Case Example: Burnout Reversed Through Quantum Hydration

A 42-year-old executive presented with fatigue, anxiety, and adrenal exhaustion. Despite drinking three liters of filtered water daily, her symptoms persisted.

She began a quantum hydration protocol:

- Switched to spring water infused with lemon and 432 Hz sound.
- Added raw cucumber and celery juice each morning.
- Charged her water daily in sunlight.
- Slept with a biophoton pillow to support intracellular coherence.

Within 10 days, she experienced:

- Clearer focus.

- Deeper sleep.
- Sustained daytime energy.

Her hydration levels hadn't changed; her water's structure had.

Summary: Water Is the Liquid Light of Life

Quantum Role of Water	Nutritional Impact
Conductor of light and frequency	Enables cellular communication.
Storage medium for biophotons	Enhances nutrient assimilation and detox.
Responsive to consciousness	Integrates intention into physiology.
Structured geometry	Optimizes hydration and energy flow.

Water is not empty. It is alive, intelligent, and essential to your light field. Structured as a liquid crystal, water becomes a nutrient of coherence, carrying the information that life itself depends on. Within each cell, water molecules align into ordered structures that respond to light, vibration, and intention, acting as a dynamic interface between matter and energy. Far beyond a passive solvent, water stores memory, transmits biophotonic signals, and orchestrates the symphony of biochemical reactions with quantum precision.

Water is the medium of life. It shapes the integrity of DNA, fuels mitochondrial energy production, and modulates the rhythms of the nervous and cardiovascular systems. When coherent, structured water amplifies vitality, enhances cellular communication, and supports the body's ability to heal itself. When disordered, it contributes to dysfunction, inflammation, and accelerated aging.

In essence, water is consciousness in motion. It is the living matrix through which biophotons travel, nourishing the body's fields with coherence and guiding the flow of information that sustains health, regeneration, and life itself.

The next chapter explores the sun as the master nutrient, the source of biophotons and biological rhythms, and how natural light sustains hormonal balance, mitochondrial vitality, and the longevity blueprint of life.

References

1. Pollack GH. The fourth phase of water: Beyond solid, liquid, and vapor. Ebner & Sons; 2013.

2. Ball, P. Water as an active constituent in cell biology. Chem Rev. 2008;108(1):74–108.

3. Del Giudice E, Tedeschi A. Water and autocatalysis in living matter. Electromagn Biol Med. 2009;28(1):46–52.

4. Zheng JM, Pollack GH. Long-range forces extending from polymer-gel surfaces. Phys Rev E. 2003;68(3):031408.

5. Cifra M, Pospíšil P. Ultra-weak photon emission and its role in living systems. J Photochem Photobiol B. 2014;139:2–10.

6. Montagnier L, Aissa J, Ferris S, Montagnier JL, Lavalléee C. Electromagnetic signals are produced by aqueous nanostructures derived from bacterial DNA sequences. Interdisciplinary Sciences: Computational Life Sciences. 2009 Jun;1(2):81–90.

7. Jonas WB, Ives JA, Rollwagen F, Denman DW, Hintz K, Hammer M, Crawford C, Henry K. Can specific biological

signals be digitized? FASEB J. 2006 Jan;20(1):23-8. doi: 10.1096/fj.05-3815hyp. PMID: 16394263.

8. Emoto M. The hidden messages in water. Beyond Words; 2004.

9. Chaplin M. Do we underestimate the importance of water structure in biological processes? Nat Rev Mol Cell Biol. 2006;7:861–866.

CHAPTER 13

Sunlight as a Master Nutrient

Feeding the Body's Photonic Economy for Energy, Hormones, and Longevity

---

The sun is not just a source of warmth—it is the original source of life's information.

—James Z. Liu, MD, PhD

Sunlight: The Forgotten Nutrient

In every seed that sprouts, every leaf that turns skyward, and every mitochondrion generating energy in your body, sunlight is present.

Sunlight is not simply environmental. It is a master nutrient delivering electromagnetic frequencies that regulate circadian rhythm, hormonal balance, immunity, and longevity [1]. Its spectrum encodes information essential for health, yet in modern life, we often block or avoid it, leaving our biophotonic systems undernourished.

Quantum nutrition restores sunlight to its rightful place: not merely as a vitamin D trigger, but as primary photonic nourishment for the human field.

Sunlight: A Spectrum of Biological Intelligence

Different wavelengths of sunlight provide distinct biological functions:

Wavelength	Range	Biological Function
UVB	280–315 nm	Stimulates vitamin D synthesis [2]
UVA	315–400 nm	Releases nitric oxide, supports immune balance, modulates mood [3]
Visible Light	400–700 nm	Entrains circadian rhythm, regulates melatonin, and balances hormones [4]
Red Light	620–750 nm	Stimulates ATP production, supports tissue repair, and stimulates stem cell activation [5]
Near-Infrared (NIR)	750–1200 nm	Penetrates deeply, structures water, enhances mitochondrial efficiency, reduces inflammation [6]

Together, this full-spectrum code provides the body with coherence and rhythm. Without it, metabolism slows, circadian signals weaken, and the biofield dims.

Sunlight as Quantum Food

Like food delivers molecules, sunlight delivers photons and frequency, feeding the biophotonic economy of life.

- Energizes mitochondria: Red and NIR light activate cytochrome c oxidase, boosting ATP output [5].
- Structures water: Infrared light charges the exclusion zone (EZ) water, enhancing detox and nutrient transport [6].
- Synchronizes circadian rhythm: Morning light through the retina resets clocks for digestion, sleep, and hormone cycles [4].
- Boosts nitric oxide: UVA dilates vessels, lowering blood pressure and supporting circulation [3].

- Supports mood and immunity: Light deficiency contributes to Seasonal Affective Disorder and immune suppression [7].

Sunlight is quantum food: energy, order, and coherence delivered at the speed of light.

Mitochondria: Solar-Powered Engines

Every cell contains hundreds to thousands of mitochondria, ancient organelles tuned to light.

Research in photobiomodulation shows that:

- Red light increases mitochondrial membrane potential.
- NIR reduces oxidative stress and enhances cellular repair [5,6].
- Cells exposed to light emit more coherent biophotons, signaling improved vitality [8].

Mitochondria are literally solar-powered batteries. Light exposure improves metabolism, cognition, endurance, and emotional resilience.

Vitamin D: Only Part of the Story

Mainstream medicine highlights vitamin D production from UVB, but this is only one fraction of sunlight's value.

Vitamin D functions as a hormone precursor, regulating more than 2,000 genes tied to immunity, inflammation, and growth [2]. But even with optimal vitamin D, the body still requires red, NIR, and visible light for mitochondrial and circadian health. No supplement can replace the photonic breadth of natural sunlight.

How Modern Living Blocks the Sun

Today, mal-illumination is widespread:

- Indoor living under artificial light.
- Sunglasses that block retinal signaling.
- Sunscreens that filter UVB but allow UVA imbalance.
- Excessive blue light exposure at night disrupts melatonin production.

Consequences include disrupted circadian rhythms, fatigue, mood disorders, hormonal imbalance, and weakened immunity [7,9].

Sunlight Protocols for Quantum Nourishment

Practice	Quantum Benefit
Morning sun (5–15 min)	Resets circadian rhythm, boosts serotonin
Midday sun (brief, bare skin)	Supports vitamin D synthesis and immunity
Barefoot grounding in sunlight	Enhances electron flow, improves light absorption
Expose food/water to the sun	Imprints solar frequencies, increases coherence
Red/NIR therapy in winter	Replaces missing frequencies, sustains mitochondrial output

Even 5–10 minutes of unfiltered sunlight daily can reset rhythms and elevate mitochondrial function.

Case Example: Reversing Seasonal Depression

A 39-year-old woman struggled with fatigue and depression every winter. Despite normal vitamin D levels, she described "a lack of inner light."

Her sunlight protocol included:

- 10 minutes of morning sunlight within 30 minutes of waking.
- Daily red-light therapy (660–850 nm).
- Drinking sun-charged water and eating sprouts exposed to natural light.
- Removing sunglasses outdoors to receive full-spectrum retinal input.

Within three weeks, her mood stabilized, energy returned, and brain fog cleared. She had reconnected with light as living medicine.

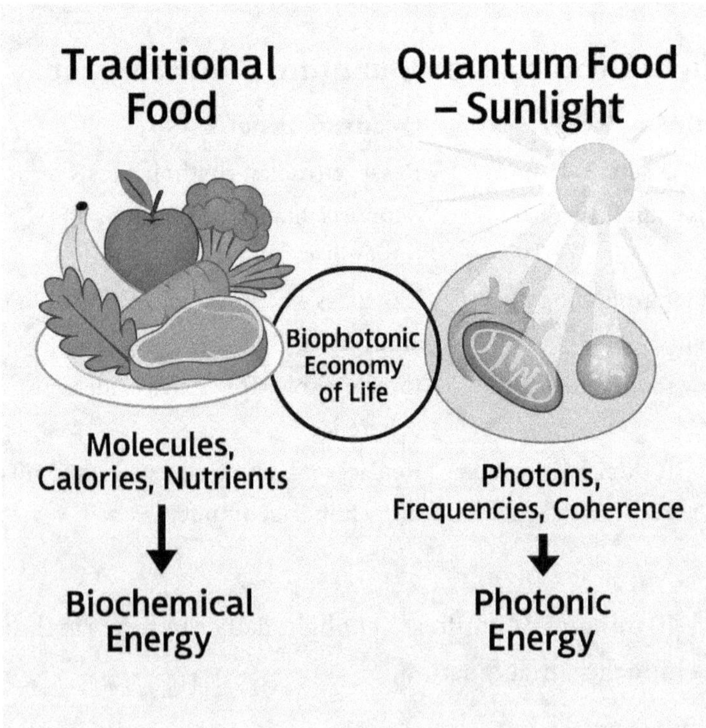

Figure 13.1. Food vs. Sunlight as Dual Sources of Nourishment. *Traditional food delivers molecules—carbohydrates, fats, proteins, and micronutrients—that fuel metabolism. Sunlight, as "quantum food," delivers photons and frequencies that feed the biophotonic economy of life, enhancing mitochondrial energy, coherence, and cellular communication. Together, both sustain human vitality.*

Summary: The Sun Is Your Original Superfood

Frequency	Function
UVB	Vitamin D synthesis, skin immunity
UVA	Nitric oxide release, mood, vascular health
Visible light	Circadian regulation, melatonin balance
Red/NIR	Mitochondrial recharging, reduced inflammation

Sunlight is not optional. It is a master nutrient, providing frequencies essential for coherence, regeneration, and vitality.

Instead of fearing the sun, quantum nutrition invites us to use it wisely, as the original source of life's information.

The next chapter will explore how to synergize photons from food, water, and sunlight, creating a daily quantum nourishment routine for regeneration, energy, and radiant health.

References

1. van Wijk R. Light in shaping Life: Biophotons in biology and medicine. Meluna Publishing; 2014.
2. Holick MF. Vitamin D deficiency. N Engl J Med. 2007;357(3):266–281.
3. Liu D, et al. UVA irradiation of human skin vasodilates arterial vasculature and lowers blood pressure. Circ Res. 2014;114(7):1083–1090.
4. Czeisler CA, et al. Bright light induction of strong (type 0) resetting of the human circadian pacemaker. Science. 1989;244(4910):1328–1333.

5. Hamblin MR. Mechanisms and applications of the anti-inflammatory effects of photobiomodulation. AIMS Biophys. 2017;4(3):337–361.
6. Pollack GH. The fourth phase of water. Ebner & Sons; 2013.
7. Rosenthal NE, et al. Seasonal affective disorder: a description of the syndrome and preliminary findings with light therapy. Arch Gen Psychiatry. 1984;41(1):72–80.
8. Tang R, Dai J. Biophoton signal transmission and biological information communication. Sci China C Life Sci. 2014;57(4):343–355.
9. Cho Y, et al. Effects of artificial light at night on human health: A literature review of observational and experimental studies. Chronobiol Int. 2015;32(9):1294–1310.

CHAPTER 14

How to Combine Biophoton Exposure

Creating a Synergistic Daily Routine for Regeneration and Vitality

---

True healing begins when the body becomes a coherent field of light. Nourish it from all directions.
—James Z. Liu, MD, PhD

The Power of Synergy

By now, we've learned that light is a nutrient, water is a conductor, food is information, and the body is a living field of frequency. But the true power of quantum nutrition does not lie in isolated practices; it emerges from synergy, when these inputs align and reinforce each other.

In quantum biology, synergy is not just efficient; it is resonant amplification. When multiple forms of biophoton nourishment interact, their effects multiply:

- A raw salad eaten under natural sunlight entrains circadian rhythm, hydrates cells, and simultaneously restores mitochondrial function [1,6].
- Red light therapy applied to a hydrated, mineral-rich body penetrates more deeply, charging structured water and enhancing energy transfer [9,3].

- A sprout grown in sunlight, eaten mindfully, and blessed with gratitude becomes a total-field alignment event, nourishing not just the body but also consciousness [10,11].

This resonance fosters greater mitochondrial output, faster detoxification and cellular turnover, stabilized emotional energy, deeper sleep and recovery, and slowed or even reversed biological aging [13,14].

The Four Pillars of Daily Biophoton Synergy

1. Sunlight: The Morning Reset

Goal: Start the day by charging your field with natural light.
Practice:

- Spend 5–15 minutes in early sun, allowing light to reach your eyes and skin.
- Stand barefoot on earth (grounding enhances electron flow).
- Drink sun-charged or lemon water before eating.

Why it works:

- Morning UVA and red/NIR light stimulate mitochondria and cortisol balance.
- Light through the retina sets circadian clocks for hormones and digestion [1].
- Grounding enhances bioelectrical conductivity [5].

2. Water: The Light Conductor

Goal: Hydrate with structured, coherent water to carry photons.
Practice:

- Drink spring, vortexed, or sun-charged water.
- Eat hydrophilic foods (cucumbers, celery, melons).

- Avoid microwaved or stagnant water; restructure if needed.

Why it works:

- Structured water forms a liquid crystal matrix that stores light [9,2].
- Increases nutrient transport and detoxification efficiency.

3. Food: The Information of Light

Goal: Eat biophoton-rich foods that transmit coherent signals.
Practice:

- Prioritize raw, organic, sun-grown produce: sprouts, greens, berries, herbs.
- Use fresh herbs, sea vegetables, and fermented foods for immune–gut resonance.
- Briefly sun-charge food before eating.
- Avoid processed or irradiated foods.

Why it works:

- Foods with intact structure emit coherent biophotons [10,12].
- Fermented foods provide rhythmic light pulses that support gut and immunity [4].

4. Biophoton Therapies: The Coherence Amplifiers

Goal: Apply intentional light therapies to boost regeneration.
Practice:

- Use red/NIR panels or Tesla BioHealers for 10–30 minutes daily on key areas (brain, chest, abdomen, joints).
- Sleep near biophoton generators or use biophoton-infused textiles.

- Pair with meditation or slow breathing to enhance absorption.

Why it works:

- Red/NIR light restores mitochondrial membrane potential and reduces inflammation [3,6].
- Nighttime light fields stabilize HRV and enhance stem cell activation [8].

A Sample Daily Biophoton Routine

Time	Activity	Quantum Impact
6:30–8:00 AM	Morning sunlight, barefoot grounding, sun-charged water	Resets circadian rhythm, charges biofield
8:00 AM	Raw fruit or green juice, gratitude practice	Provides coherent food information
12:00 PM	Midday sun + fresh salad with fermented veggies	Boosts vitamin D, immune coherence
3:00 PM	Structured water, herbal tea, and a brief outdoor walk	Sustains hydration and photon flow
6:00 PM	Light dinner: sprouted grains, steamed greens	Gentle nourishment maintains coherence
8:00 PM	Red/NIR therapy or biophoton generator (15–30 min)	Mitochondrial repair, anti-inflammatory effects
10:00 PM	Sleep with a biophoton pillow or mat; structured water nearby	Enhances recovery, stem cell activation

This template is adaptable, but consistency of light, water, food, and intention allows the body to become entrained into a rhythm of coherence and regeneration.

Healing Happens in Layers

Biophoton synergy rewires cellular communication gradually, not overnight.

- First few days: better sleep, sharper focus, deeper hydration.
- 1–2 weeks: mood uplift, more energy, improved digestion.
- 30+ days: skin radiance, stable hormones, deeper recovery cycles.
- Long-term: slowed biological aging, improved resilience, greater intuitive clarity.

This is quantum regeneration: building health at the field level, not just masking symptoms.

Case Example: Chronic Inflammation Transformed

A 60-year-old man with arthritis and metabolic syndrome adopted a daily synergy plan:

- Green smoothies with raw sprouts.
- Sun-charged, structured water each morning.
- 15 minutes of red-light therapy on joints.
- Sleeping with a biophoton pillow.
- Cutting microwaved foods and processed snacks.

Results after two weeks:

- Reduced joint pain and inflammation.
- Five pounds of weight loss without added exercise.

- Restored morning energy and digestive regularity.
- Improved sleep quality and emotional balance.

His physician noted improved markers, without the need for new medications. His transformation came from field coherence, not pharmacology.

Summary: Stack the Light, Heal the Field

Biophoton Source	Key Action
Sunlight	Resets circadian and mitochondrial cycles.
Structured Water	Enhances photon flow and hydration.
Raw Food	Provides coherent information for regulation.
Light Therapy	Amplifies repair, regeneration, and sleep.

When the body's field synchronizes across systems, light, water, food, and breath become a single song of resonance. This is the foundation of lasting vitality.

The next chapter will explore how to measure progress using biological age, biofield coherence, mitochondrial output, and non-invasive photonic biomarkers to track the evolution of your inner light [3].

References

1. Cajochen, C., Zeitzer, J. M., Czeisler, C. A., & Dijk, D. J. Dose-response relationship for light intensity and ocular melatonin suppression in humans. *Journal of Physiology*. 2000;549(3):963–970.

2. Fritz, G. J. Structured water, health, and longevity: A biophysical perspective. *Water Journal.* 2019;11:1–15.

3. Hamblin, M. R., & Demidova, T. N. (2006). Mechanisms of low-level light therapy. In *Mechanisms for Low-Light Therapy.* 2006;6140:614001. SPIE. doi:10.1117/12.646294

4. Baskerville R. et al. The effect of photobiomodulation on the treatment of hereditary mitochondrial diseases. *J Lasers Med Sci.* 2023 Oct 10;14:e41. doi: 10.34172/jlms.2023.41

5. Jerman, I., Ružič, R., Krašovec, R., & Leskovar, R. T. Bioelectromagnetic communication within living systems: Theoretical and experimental aspects. *Electromagnetic Biology and Medicine.* 2009;28(1):84–99.

6. Karu, T. I. Multiple roles of cytochrome c oxidase in mammalian cells under action of red and infrared light. *IUBMB Life.* 2010;62(8):607–610. doi:10.1002/iub.359

7. Su CT and Wu JH. Photobiomodulation in biological tissues: Light penetration, dosimetry, and potential applications. *Optics and Lasers in Engineering.* 2025 March;186:108852.

8. Smotrys MA, Gu HY, Poirier LJ, Ager A, JZ Liu JZ. Biophoton therapy enhances endogenous stem-cell production: A non-Invasive approach to regenerative medicine. *J Neurol Res Rev Rep.* 2025;7(12):1-11.

9. Pollack, G. H. *The fourth phase of water: Beyond solid, liquid, and vapor.* Ebner and Sons Publishers; 2013.

10. Popp, F. A., Gurwitsch, A. G., Rattemeyer, M., Schäfer, F., & Walleczek, J. Biophoton emission: Experimental background and theoretical approaches. *Modern Physics Letters B.* 1988;2(05):831–840.

11. Rubik, B., Muehsam, D., Hammerschlag, R., & Jain, S. Biofield science and healing: History, terminology, and concepts. *Global Advances in Health and Medicine.* 2015;4(Suppl 1):8–14. doi:10.7453/gahmj.2015.038.suppl

12. van Wijk, E. P. A., van Wijk, R., & Bajpai, R. P. Ultraweak photon emission of the human body. *Indian Journal of Experimental Biology*. 2006;44(5):358–362.

13. Uttke, W., et al. Photobiomodulation and mitochondrial function: Light at the end of the tunnel. *Trends in Biochemical Sciences.* 2018;43(6):406–419.

14. Bajpai RP. Quantum coherence of biophotons and living systems. *Indian J Exp Biol.* 2003 May;41(5):514–27.

CHAPTER 15

How to Measure Progress and Biological Age Reversal

Tracking Regeneration Through Biophoton Markers, Biofield Coherence, and Non-Invasive Tools

---

If you can measure the light within, you can measure your return to youth.
—James Z. Liu, MD, PhD

The promise of quantum nutrition extends beyond more energy, deeper sleep, and emotional balance. Its most exciting potential is the reversal of biological age.

Chronological age is fixed, but biological age—the functional status of your cells and tissues—can move in either direction. With the right inputs, biological age can be slowed, paused, or even reversed [1,2].

New tools from biophysics, photomedicine, and integrative diagnostics now allow us to track regeneration not by weight or calories, but by light [4–6].

Quantum metrics of progress include:

- Biophoton emission,
- Biofield coherence,
- Mitochondrial performance,

- Biological age algorithms,
- Heart rate variability (HRV) and subtle energy markers.

These measures allow you to see and optimize your healing trajectory as your body's light field strengthens.

What Is Biological Age?

Biological age reflects the functional state of the body and is shaped by:

- DNA methylation and gene expression patterns [1]
- Inflammation and oxidative stress [2]
- Mitochondrial energy output [3]
- Cellular repair and regeneration rate [2,3]
- Hormonal and immune balance [2]

Unlike chronological age, biological age is dynamic. A 60-year-old may function biologically as a 45-year-old—or, conversely, a 35-year-old under stress, a poor diet, or a photon deficiency may test as decades "older" [2].

Quantum nutrition restores coherence in the body's light field, creating conditions for renewal [4,6].

Biophoton Emission: Light as a Vitality Marker

All living cells emit ultraweak photons, known as biophotons. Their intensity and coherence mirror cellular health and vitality [4,6].

How it is measured:

- Photomultiplier tubes or ultrasensitive CCD cameras [4]
- Gas Discharge Visualization (GDV)/Bio-Well fingertip scans [5]
- Mapping photon emissions from skin or organs [6]

What it reveals:

- Strong, coherent light → vitality, regeneration, and systemic alignment [4,6]
- Weak or chaotic light → inflammation, stress, accelerated aging [6]

Clinical studies show that biophoton emissions rise with raw foods, red light therapy, and structured water [6–8]. Tracking photon output over time provides a quantum biomarker of rejuvenation.

Biofield Coherence: The Rhythm of Regeneration

The biofield is the body's endogenous electromagnetic field. When coherent, it signals harmony; when fragmented, it signals imbalance [5,10].

How it is measured:

- HRV: heart rate variability reflects autonomic nervous system tone [9]
- Bio-Well/GDV scans: visualize field strength and symmetry [5]
- EEG/ECG coherence: measure alignment of brain and heart rhythms [10]

Benefits of improved coherence:

- Deeper sleep and faster recovery [10]
- Reduced stress reactivity [9,10]
- Enhanced immunity [2,10]
- Slower biological aging [1,2,9]

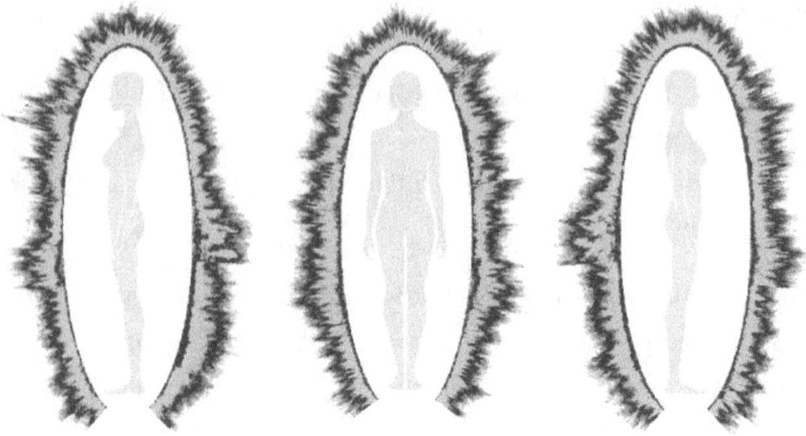

Figure 15.1. ***A Healthy Human Body with a Perfect Aura.*** *Illustration of a healthy human body surrounded by a vibrant and coherent biofield. The radiant, symmetrical aura signifies balanced energy flow, strong vitality, and optimal well-being.*

Benefits of improved coherence:

- Deeper sleep and faster recovery,
- Reduced stress reactivity,
- Enhanced immunity,
- Slower biological aging.

A more stable HRV and field signature indicate your system is moving toward regeneration.

Mitochondrial Performance

Mitochondria are the "power plants" of cells and are central to aging. When mitochondrial efficiency declines, energy drops, inflammation rises, and cellular decay accelerates [2,3].

Assessing mitochondrial health:

- ATP output (organic acids, bioenergetic panels) [3]

- Lactate/Pyruvate ratios (energy pathway efficiency) [3]
- VO_2 max and post-exercise recovery [3]
- Subjective markers: stamina, focus, muscle recovery [3]

Photon-rich interventions, including red light therapy, structured water, and nutrient-dense raw foods, recharge mitochondrial membranes and often improve measurable metrics within weeks [7,8].

Red light therapy, structured water, and photon-rich foods directly recharge mitochondrial membranes, often improving metrics within weeks [3].

Biological Age Calculators and Tests

Method	What It Measures	Quantum Relevance
DNA methylation (e.g., TruAge)	Epigenetic "gene expression age"	Long-term changes, validates sustained coherence.
Telomere length (TeloYears)	Cellular division potential	Slower to change but shows regeneration over years.
Heart Rate Variability (HRV)	Nervous system and biofield tone	Rapidly reflects hydration, breath, and light practices.
Bio-Well/GDV Imaging	Biophoton symmetry and field balance	Direct measure of light-based health.
Facial/skin imaging	Collagen, circulation, microvascular age	Quick visual feedback from a photon-rich lifestyle.

For the best insight, combine molecular, field-based, and photonic tools.

Self-Assessment: Signals of Progress

You don't need lab equipment to track improvements. Week by week, notice:

- ☑ More morning energy without caffeine.
- ☑ Reduced inflammation or puffiness.
- ☑ Faster healing and recovery after exertion.
- ☑ Brighter skin, eyes, and mood.
- ☑ Sharper focus, deeper intuition, and calmer emotions.
- ☑ Improved sleep cycles and vivid dreams.
- ☑ Digestive ease and fewer food sensitivities.

These shifts reflect cellular and systemic reorganization around coherence [2,6,10].

Case Example: 65-Year-Old Woman Reverses 8 Biological Years

A 65-year-old woman began a quantum nutrition routine:

- Daily Tesla BioHealer sessions + red light exposure
- Structured spring water with lemon
- Raw living foods and fermented greens
- Sunrise light (10 minutes daily)
- Gratitude rituals before meals

After 180 days:

- Bio-Well scans → 32% increase in coherence [5]
- HRV → 25% improvement [9]
- Weight → 10 lb. decrease
- Skin brightened, sleep normalized, mood stabilized
- Epigenetic test → reversal of 8 biological years [1]

Her rejuvenation was not driven by pharmaceuticals but by light, coherence, and intention [4–7,10].

Summary: If You Track the Light, You Track the Healing

Quantum Marker	What It Tracks	Optimized By
Biophoton Emission	Cellular vitality, coherence	Raw food, light, structured water, breathwork
Biofield Imaging/HRV	Nervous system and field balance	Meditation, grounding, gratitude, hydration
Mitochondrial Performance	Energy and metabolism	Red/NIR light, structured water, movement
Biological Age Algorithms	System-wide resilience	Long-term lifestyle coherence

You are light in biological form. Your health is your frequency. And your youth is not fixed; it is measurable, reversible, and restorable.

The next chapter looks to the future: how quantum nutrition is reshaping medicine itself. We'll explore how AI, personalized light therapies, and biofield mapping are converging to form a new standard of longevity care—one rooted in light.

References

1. Horvath S, Raj K. DNA methylation-based biomarkers and the epigenetic clock theory of ageing. *Nat Rev Genet.* 2018;19(6):371–384. doi:10.1038/s41576-018-0004-3

2. López-Otín C, et al. The hallmarks of aging. *Cell.* 2013;153(6):1194–1217. doi:10.1016/j.cell.2013.05.039

3. Wallace DC. Mitochondrial genetic medicine. *Nat Genet.* 2018;50(12):1642–1649. doi:10.1038/s41588-018-0264-z

4. Popp FA. Biophoton emission: Experimental background and theoretical approaches. *Modern Physics Letters B.* 1994;8(21-22):1269-1296.

5. Korotkov K. *Human energy field: Study with GDV bioelectrography*. Fair Lawn: Backbone Publishing; 2002.

6. Salari V et al. Imaging ultraweak photon emission from living and dead mice and from plants under stress. *BioRxiv preprint.* 2024. doi:10.1101/2024.11.08.622743.

7. Hamblin MR. Mechanisms and applications of the anti-inflammatory effects of photobiomodulation. *AIMS Biophys.* 2017;4(3):337–361.

8. Giudice ED et al. The origin and the special role of coherent water in living systems. *Fields of the Cell.* 2015;95–111.

9. Shaffer F, Ginsberg JP. An overview of heart rate variability metrics and norms. *Front Public Health.* 2017;5:258. doi:10.3389/fpubh.2017.00258

10. McCraty R, Childre D. Coherence: bridging personal, social, and global health. *Altern Ther Health Med.* 2010;16(4):10–24.

11. Aubert G. and Lansdorp P. Telomeres and aging. *Physiol Rev.* 2008 Apr;88(2):557–579.

CHAPTER 16

How Biophotonic Medicine May Reshape Aging, Longevity Clinics, AI-Assisted Diagnostics, and Global Wellness Systems

The Future of Healthcare Begins with Light

The medicine of the future will be the medicine of frequencies. **—Attributed to Albert Einstein**

We stand at the dawn of a profound transformation in medicine: a move from molecular-based intervention to field-based regeneration, from symptom control to energetic coherence, and from disease management to lifespan and healthspan extension through light.

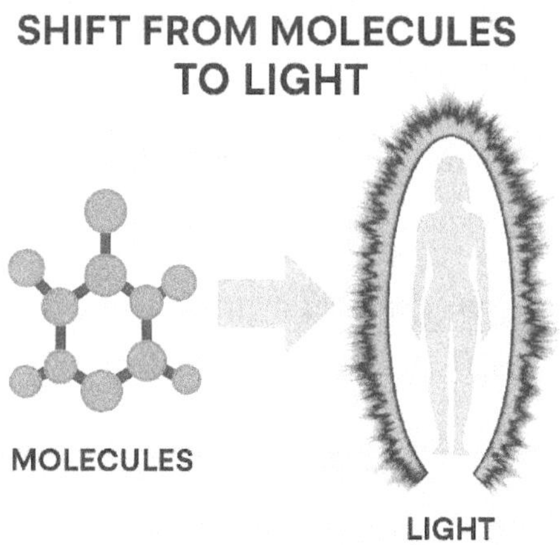

Figure 16.1. Medicine Shifts from Molecules to Light. *Illustration of the paradigm shift from molecular biology to light-based biology. The left panel represents traditional molecular structures, while the right panel shows a human figure surrounded by a radiant aura, symbolizing the transition toward understanding health and vitality through light and biofield coherence.*

Quantum nutrition is not just a personal wellness strategy; it is the foundation of biophotonic medicine in which healthcare begins not with a pill or a lab panel, but with a map of your body's light field, mitochondrial vitality, circadian synchrony, and biofield resonance.

This chapter explores how quantum nutrition converges with:

- Regenerative medicine,
- AI-assisted diagnostics,
- Non-invasive field imaging,
- Personalized phototherapy, and
- Global longevity systems.

Together, these innovations will redefine our understanding of aging, immunity, energy, and consciousness, ushering in a planetary upgrade in healthcare.

Biophotonic Medicine: From Chemistry to Coherence

Biophotonic medicine rests on three core insights:

1. Every cell emits and responds to ultra-weak photons [1].
2. Disease arises from the loss of electromagnetic coherence [2].
3. Healing occurs when the body is restored to resonance and order [3].

Instead of only correcting chemical imbalances, biophotonic medicine will:

- Map the body's light emissions and field dynamics,
- Deliver coherent inputs (red/NIR, UV, structured water, biophoton devices),
- Integrate food, water, breath, sound, and intention as energetic therapies.

It is non-invasive, personalized, data-rich, and consciousness-compatible.

The Longevity Clinic of the Future

Tomorrow's longevity clinics will look less like hospitals and more like light sanctuaries designed to realign the biophotonic ecosystem.

Core features may include:

- Biofield scanning rooms using gas discharge visualization (GDV), HRV, and coherence monitors [4].
- Photonic food bars serving biophoton-rich, enzyme-active meals [5].
- Therapy suites with red/NIR beds, Tesla BioHealers, and pulsed EMF mats [6].
- Sunlight gardens for circadian recalibration and grounding.
- Quantum hydration stations offering vortexed, mineralized, and structured water [7].
- Breath-frequency chambers combining coherent sound and intention to regulate nervous system rhythms [8].

The key clinical question will no longer be, *"What is wrong with me?"* but rather, *"Where is my light blocked and how do I restore it?"*

AI-Assisted Diagnostics and Biofield Imaging

Artificial intelligence is rapidly enhancing diagnostics. Already, AI can detect illness from voice tone, facial microexpressions, retinal images, and ECG signals [9]. These are expressions of field disruption.

In the quantum clinic of the future, AI will:

- Analyze biophoton emission patterns in real time [10],

- Predict coherence breakdowns before symptoms arise,
- Recommend personalized combinations of light, food, and breath,
- Track daily field dynamics and adapt care plans dynamically.

Paired with non-invasive biofield imaging, AI will enable diagnostics to be preventive, precise, and personalized.

Education: From Calories to Frequencies

Medical and nutrition education will also evolve. Just as practitioners today learn macronutrients, future clinicians will study:

- Photonic density of food and its coherence potential [5],
- Structured water as a medium for cellular signaling [7],
- Field entrainment techniques using light, sound, breath, and intention [8],
- Epigenetic pathways responsive to photons and vibration [11],
- Field-based biomarkers for wellness tracking [4].

Biophotonics will become a shared language among physicians, nutritionists, therapists, and mental health providers, each working with frequencies to restore coherence.

Global Biophotonic Infrastructure

For biophotonic medicine to become mainstream, accessibility is key and requires:

- Home-use tools: affordable red/NIR panels, wearable photon patches, structured water kits.
- Community wellness centers: grounding mats, infrared saunas, coherent light therapy spaces.
- Rural solar clinics: delivering light-based healing powered by solar energy.

- Tele-photonic care: remote diagnostics and phototherapy prescriptions via field scans.

Because light is universal, biophotonic healing can cross economic, geographic, and cultural boundaries.

Redefining Aging as Reversible

The greatest promise of biophotonic medicine is its ability to redefine aging.

From a field perspective, aging is not merely the passage of time, but the progressive loss of cellular coherence, mitochondrial rhythm, and biofield order [12]. These qualities are measurable and reversible.

With consistent quantum inputs, individuals can:

- Reverse biological age by 5–10+ years [13],
- Reactivate dormant stem cell pathways [14],
- Regenerate tissues and improve memory [15],
- Sustain libido, energy, and clarity into advanced age [16].

Longevity will no longer mean simply surviving longer but glowing longer.

Case Vision: A Visit to a Biophotonic Longevity Center (Year 2035)

Imagine walking into a center designed like a living organism, with flowing water and sunlight. There is no clipboard. Instead, a field scan greets you. A camera maps your photon emissions, hydration, mitochondrial pulse, and biofield coherence.

Within minutes, AI generates your light map and prescribes:

- A personalized phototherapy plan,

- A vibrational food schedule,
- A coherent water regimen,
- A breath-and-movement protocol,
- A sleep module inside a biophoton cocoon.

No drugs. No invasive procedures. Just resonance restoration. And each day, your metrics and your vitality rise.

Summary: A Global Shift Begins with a Photon

Element	Transformation Through Biophotons
Medicine	From lab tests → field imaging and light-based healing
Nutrition	From calories → photonic information and coherence
Diagnostics	From invasive scans → AI + real-time energy analytics
Aging	From decline → measurable regeneration
Global Wellness	From fragmented care → universal light access

The next revolution will not come in syringes or surgeries. It will come in sunlight, sprouts, structured water, coherent breath, and intention, delivered with precision, intelligence, and compassion.

References

1. Popp FA, et al. Biophoton emission: New evidence for coherence in living biological systems. In: *Electromagnetic Bio-Information.* Urban & Schwarzenberg; 1981.

2. Bischof M. Biophotons: The light in our cells. *J Opt Phototherapy.* 2005;13(1):2–6.

3. Van Wijk R, Van Wijk EP. Biophotons and bio-communication. *J Sci Explor.* 2005;19(4):531–545.

4. Rubik B. The biofield hypothesis: Its biophysical basis and role in medicine. *J Altern Complement Med.* 2002;8(6):703–717.

5. Fels D. Cellular communication through light. *PLoS ONE.* 2009;4(4):e5086.

6. Hamblin MR. Mechanisms and applications of photobiomodulation. *AIMS Biophys.* 2017;4(3):337–361.

7. Pollack GH. *The fourth phase of water: Beyond solid, liquid, and vapor.* Ebner & Sons; 2013.

8. Tiller WA. *Science and human transformation.* Pavior Publishing; 1997.

9. Schuller BW, et al. Emotionally adaptive support: a narrative review of affective computing for mental health. *Front. Digit. Health.* 2025;7.

10. Tang R, Dai J. Biophoton signal transmission and biological information communication. *Sci China C Life Sci.* 2014;57(4):343–355.

11. Albrecht-Buehler G. Cell intelligence: communication and decision-making. *Trends Cell Biol.* 1992;2(3):81–84.

12. López-Otín C, et al. The hallmarks of aging. *Cell.* 2013;153(6):1194–1217.

13. Fahy GM, et al. Reversal of epigenetic aging and immunosenescent trends in humans. *Aging Cell.* 2019;18(6):e13028.

14. Weissman IL. Stem cells: units of development, units of regeneration, units in evolution. *Cell.* 2000;100(1):157–168.

15. Ma Q. Role of Nrf2 in oxidative stress and toxicity. *Annu Rev Pharmacol Toxicol.* 2013;53:401–426.

16. Rosenthal NE, et al. Seasonal affective disorder and light therapy. *Arch Gen Psychiatry*. 1984;41(1):72–80.

CHAPTER 17

Deglycation and Detox with Quantum Inputs

Anti-Aging and Anti-Inflammatory Mechanisms Through Light, Water, and Field Coherence

---

Aging begins with entanglement—when proteins, sugars, and toxins lose rhythm. But light reintroduces order. —**James Z. Liu, MD, PhD**

Aging as the Accumulation of Error

Aging is not simply the passage of years; it is the accumulation of molecular errors and energetic disarray. Over time, disordered proteins, toxic residues, and metabolic misfires dim the body's biophotonic field. Two of the most damaging contributors are:

- Glycation of sugars to proteins, lipids, or DNA, producing advanced glycation end-products (AGEs).
- Toxic accumulation: heavy metals, plastics, synthetic chemicals, and metabolic wastes that disrupt coherence.

Both processes stiffen tissues, fuel inflammation, and erode mitochondrial vitality [1,2]. Quantum nutrition reframes anti-aging not as chemical warfare against each molecule, but as restoring order, light, and field coherence through biophotonic inputs.

Part I: Understanding Glycation: The "Caramelization" of Aging

Glycation is a non-enzymatic reaction where sugars bind to proteins, lipids, or DNA. The resulting AGEs:

- Crosslink collagen → wrinkles, loss of elasticity.
- Harden arteries → cardiovascular stiffness.
- Accumulate in the brain → Alzheimer's plaques.
- Damage kidneys and retina.
- Impair cellular repair and energy metabolism [3,4].

In essence, glycation is akin to internal rusting, a sticky entropy that clogs life's rhythm.

How Quantum Inputs Reverse Glycation

1. Red and Near-Infrared (NIR) Light

- Penetrates tissue and stimulates cytochrome c oxidase, boosting ATP production.
- Enhances enzymes that repair or degrade cross-linked proteins.
- Improves circulation to flush AGE byproducts [5,6].
- Studies show that light at 660–850 nm reduces oxidative stress and protein misfolding [7].

2. Biophoton-Rich Raw Foods

- Supply enzymes and antioxidants (e.g., carnosine, sulforaphane, quercetin) that block AGE formation.
- Sprouts, berries, turmeric, garlic, and chlorophyll-rich greens reduce glycation pathways [8].

3. Structured Water

- Forms exclusion zone (EZ) lattices that stabilize protein folding [9].
- Improves enzymatic activity and flexibility, reducing aggregation.
- Helps cells "uncouple" glycated proteins from receptors.

4. Coherence Restoration via the Biofield

- Strong, coherent biofields accelerate repair and resist entropic glycation.
- Field synchronization fosters resilience across tissues [10].

In sum:

- Light loosens sticky bonds.
- Water flushes debris.
- Food supplies repair codes.
- Coherence keeps the system resilient.

Part II: Quantum Detox: Clearing the Biofield Burden

Toxins are not just chemicals; they are **frequency disruptors** that interfere with cellular signaling and photon flow.

Common quantum-interfering toxins:

- Heavy metals (mercury, cadmium, lead)
- Plastics (BPA, phthalates)
- Agricultural chemicals (glyphosate)
- Mold mycotoxins
- Electromagnetic pollution (non-native EMFs) [11,12]

These toxins suppress mitochondria, disrupt hormones, inflame neurons, and fragment the biofield.

Quantum Detox Strategies

1. Sunlight and Red Light Detox

- Stimulates lymphatic flow and mitophagy (damaged mitochondria clearance).
- Increases intracellular charge, aiding toxin release [5,6].

2. Structured Water + Electrolytes

- Promotes urinary and sweat elimination.
- Restores negative charge to tissues.
- Helps dissolve biofilm-bound toxins [9].

3. High Fiber, Enzyme-Rich Foods

- Bind toxins in the gut.
- Feed microbiota that produce glutathione and detox enzymes.
- Foods like chia, flax, spirulina, and fermented fibers support gut–field detox [13].

4. Grounding and Breathwork

- Transfers Earth's free electrons, neutralizing oxidative stress.
- Deep breathing increases vagal tone, opening detox pathways [14].

5. Biophoton Field Activation (e.g., Tesla BioHealers)

- Floods the system with coherent light.
- Resets immune coordination and DNA repair enzymes.
- Supports nighttime detox and regeneration [15].

Case Example: 30-Day Quantum Deglycation Protocol

A 58-year-old man with joint pain, brain fog, and facial aging began:

- Raw greens and anti-glycation foods (turmeric, berries).
- 20 minutes of red-light therapy daily.
- Tesla BioHealer was placed near his liver area at night.
- 3 liters/day of structured water with minerals.
- Morning barefoot sun-walks and breathwork.

Results after 30 days:

- 70% reduction in joint pain.
- Brighter skin and clearer eyes.
- Lost 6 lbs. of inflammatory bloat.
- Improved memory and libido.
- HRV rose by 22%; biofield imaging showed increased coherence.

The light didn't just clear toxins—it restored his field identity.

Anti-Inflammation Through Coherence

Chronic inflammation is not only biochemical; it is a loss of order. When mitochondria are sluggish, water is unstructured, and the biofield frays, cells signal "danger" endlessly. The results:

- Autoimmune flares,
- Sleep disruption,
- Accelerated aging,
- Emotional instability [16].

Quantum inputs reintroduce rhythm. Cells begin to trust their environment again, and inflammatory chaos gives way to calm coherence.

Summary: Deglycation and Detox Are Energetic First, Chemical Second

Quantum Tool	Deglycation Effect	Detox Effect
Red/NIR Light	Breaks crosslinks, repairs proteins	Mitochondrial clearance, lymphatic flow
Structured Water	Improves enzyme flexibility	Flushes toxins, stabilizes charge
Raw Plant Foods	Antioxidants, anti-glycation compounds	Fiber binding, microbiome support
Biophoton Therapies	Restores DNA repair and coherence	Field-based detox, immune regulation
Grounding + Breathwork	Enhances parasympathetic tone	EMF/cortisol reduction, polarity restored

Deglycation is not just chemical; it is repatterning the geometry of light.

Detox is not just elimination; it is unburdening the field so regeneration can begin.

Quantum inputs offer a unified approach to anti-aging, working from both the inside and the outside.

References

1. Brownlee M. Advanced protein glycosylation in diabetes and aging. *Annu Rev Med.* 1995;46:223–234.
2. Vistoli G, et al. Advanced glycoxidation and lipoxidation end products (AGEs and ALEs). *Free Radic Biol Med.* 2013;65:1057–1065.

3. Ott C, et al. Role of advanced glycation end products in cellular signaling. *Redox Biol.* 2014;2:411–429.

4. Srikanth V, et al. Advanced glycation endproducts and their relevance in aging. *Curr Aging Sci.* 2011;4(3):248–259.

5. Hamblin MR. Mechanisms and applications of the anti-inflammatory effects of photobiomodulation. *AIMS Biophys.* 2017;4(3):337–361.

6. Salehpour F, et al. Therapeutic potential of intranasal photobiomodulation therapy. *J Photochem Photobiol B.* 2019;194:1–23.

7. Moro, C., El Massri, N., Torres, N., Ratel, D., De Jaeger, X., Chabrol, C., et al. Photobiomodulation inside the brain: a novel method of applying near-infrared light intracranially and its impact on dopaminergic cell survival in MPTP-treated mice. *J. Neurosurg.* 2014;120:670–683.

8. Hipkiss AR. Carnosine and its possible roles in nutrition and health. *Adv Food Nutr Res.* 2009;57:87–154.

9. Pollack GH. *The fourth phase of water: Beyond solid, liquid, and vapor.* Ebner & Sons; 2013.

10. Rubik B. The biofield hypothesis: Its biophysical basis and role in medicine. *J Altern Complement Med.* 2002;8(6):703–717.

11. Miller GW, Jones DP. The nature of nurture: refining the toxic exposome. *Toxicol Sci.* 2014;137(1):1–2.

12. Valko M, et al. Metals, toxicity and oxidative stress. *Curr Med Chem.* 2005;12(10):1161–1208.

13. Deehan EC, Walter J. The fiber gap and the disappearing gut microbiome. *Nutrients.* 2016;8(9):625.

14. Chevalier G, et al. Earthing: health implications of reconnecting the human body to the Earth's surface electrons. *J Environ Public Health.* 2012;2012:291541.

15. Popp FA, Gu Q and KH LI. Biophoton emission: experimental background and theoretical approaches. *Modern Physics Letters B.* 1994;8(21-22):1269-1296.

16. López-Otín C, et al. The hallmarks of aging. *Cell.* 2013;153(6):1194–1217.

PART III

Practical Quantum Nutrition

Part III transitions from theory to practice, providing concrete strategies for applying biophoton science in everyday life. These chapters demonstrate that quantum nutrition is not just a concept, but a lived reality—one that can transform health, longevity, and even our relationship with the world around us.

Chapter 18 provides guidance on *building a biophoton-rich diet,* prioritizing fresh, raw, and light-infused foods that carry the highest levels of coherent energy.

Chapter 19 expands into *quantum meal planning,* offering practical frameworks for designing meals that harmonize light, structure, and frequency for optimal cellular vitality.

Chapter 20 explores how to *integrate biophoton devices,* from red/near-infrared light to Tesla BioHealers, into daily routines for sustained energy and regenerative outcomes.

Chapter 21 demonstrates how pets, with their heightened sensitivity to energy, benefit profoundly from *quantum nutrition,* showing measurable improvements in vitality, mobility, and emotional balance.

Chapter 22 extends the discussion to *plants,* highlighting how structured water, photonic cultivation, and coherent environments increase yield, resilience, and nutrient density.

Chapter 23 applies quantum nutrition to *medicine and longevity,* presenting emerging protocols for reversing biological aging, restoring coherence, and managing chronic disease through light-based therapies.

Chapter 24 looks ahead to *AI and frequency mapping*, envisioning a future where biofield scans, quantum biomarkers, and personalized algorithms create individualized nutrition plans tuned to one's vibrational needs.

Chapter 25 challenges the foundations of conventional healthcare by *rewriting the human health paradigm* from disease management to coherence cultivation across body, mind, and society.

Chapter 26 offers a lived philosophy of *being a quantum being*, emphasizing practices of coherence, rhythm, and conscious nourishment that extend beyond food to daily life.

Chapter 27 reframes *mitochondrial deficiency as biophoton deficiency*, showing how fatigue, degeneration, and chronic conditions are rooted in lost cellular light.

Chapter 28 closes this section by arguing that *biophoton deficiency and lack of coherence underlie the most common modern disorders*, positioning quantum nutrition as a primary path to prevention and healing.

Together, these chapters form a practical roadmap for embodying quantum nutrition. They show how light-based nourishment can be applied not only to diet, but to pets, plants, medicine, and society, bridging personal vitality with planetary coherence.

CHAPTER 18

Building a Biophoton-Rich Diet

Foods, Habits, and Cooking Methods That Preserve Light

Eat food that still remembers the sun.

—James Z. Liu, MD, PhD

Beyond Calories: Food as Light Information

In quantum nutrition, food is more than protein, carbohydrates, or fat. It is a living messenger, encoded with biophotons: ultraweak, coherent light emitted by all living organisms.

These emissions are not random. They correlate with cellular order, vitality, and immune resilience [1,2]. Dr. Fritz-Albert Popp's pioneering research demonstrated that fresh, unprocessed foods with higher photon emissions enhance intercellular communication, mitochondrial efficiency, and DNA repair. In contrast, processed foods emit weaker or chaotic light [3,4].

Thus, the goal of a biophoton-rich diet is to nourish the body with photonic intelligence, light that cells can absorb, use, and resonate with.

What Is Biophoton-Rich Food?

Biophoton-rich foods are those that emit strong, coherent ultraweak light, measurable with photomultiplier tubes and CCD cameras [5]. Their light originates from: (1) Photosynthesis: sunlight stored as molecular order in plants. (2) High enzymatic activity: live metabolic processes. (3) Ordered cellular structure: intact membranes and cytoskeletons. (4) Living water: structured intracellular water that conducts bioinformation [6].

Top Biophoton-Rich Foods

Category	Examples
Raw Greens and Sprouts	Broccoli sprouts, sunflower sprouts, wheatgrass, kale, arugula
Berries and Fruits	Wild blueberries, blackberries, pomegranate, papaya, mango (sun-ripened)
Living Seeds and Nuts	Soaked flax, chia, pumpkin seeds, sprouted almonds and walnuts
Fermented Foods	Raw sauerkraut, kimchi, kefir, kombucha, miso
Herbs and Wild Plants	Cilantro, basil, parsley, nettle, dandelion greens
Sea Vegetables	Dulse, kelp, nori, Irish moss

Note: Freshness matters. Photon emissions decline rapidly after harvest and storage [3,7].

Storage Habits That Preserve Light

1. Buy local and seasonal. Shorter supply chains = higher photon retention [8].
2. Avoid prolonged refrigeration. Cold slows decay but also dims photon activity. Store greens in breathable containers or a damp cloth.

3. Wash just before eating. Washing early can disrupt microbiota and surface light patterns.
4. Avoid plastics. Store in glass, ceramic, or paper to maintain vibrational integrity [9].

Cooking: Preserve the Light, Don't Kill It

Cooking alters not only enzymes but also photonic coherence. Excessive heat, microwaving, and frying degrade biophoton emissions [10].

Best methods for preserving light:

Method	Why It Works
Steaming	Retains water structure and many phytonutrients while softening fibers
Low-heat sautéing (<118°F / 47°C)	Preserves enzymes and antioxidant compounds
Slow cooking with hydration	Maintains structure if consumed fresh with herbs
Sun-drying/sun-charging	Concentrates and preserves photon content if done naturally

Avoid: Microwaving, deep frying, and high-heat grilling create incoherent light signatures and oxidative byproducts [10,11].

Daily Habits to Increase Your Dietary Light

1. Sun-charge your food. Place fruits, herbs, or water in sunlight for 10–30 minutes [12].
2. Bless your meals. Intention and gratitude increase the coherence of food's water crystals [13].

3. Eat with presence. Avoid distractions; coherence in the eater amplifies coherence in the food [14].
4. Grow something fresh. Even a tray of sprouts provides the highest photon density per gram [7].
5. Chew slowly. Enzyme activation and photonic signaling begin in the mouth.

Sample One-Day Biophoton-Rich Meal Plan

Time	Meal
Morning	Sun-charged cucumber–celery juice + soaked chia seeds + breathwork in sunlight
Breakfast	Fresh papaya with lime, sprouted buckwheat groats, and raw honey drizzle
Lunch	Raw kale–avocado salad with fermented carrots, sunflower sprouts, olive oil, lemon
Snack	Sun-dried nettle or tulsi tea + soaked walnuts and wild blueberries
Dinner	Lightly steamed greens, fermented brown rice, miso broth with seaweed and cilantro
Night	Structured water + red/NIR light or biophoton pillow session

This plan supports hydration, mitochondrial repair, detoxification, and field coherence.

Advanced Strategies for Light Nutrition

- Grow your own microgreens: 7–10 days from seed to harvest = maximal photon emission [7].
- Include chlorophyll daily: Transfers solar energy directly into mitochondrial activity [15].

- Pair raw meals with red light therapy: Enhances assimilation and ATP production [5,6].
- Cook with structured water: Transmits vibrational information into soups, teas, and grains [9].

Summary: Eat the Light That Builds the Field

Biophoton Principle	Practical Strategy
Coherent foods → coherent cells	Prioritize raw, local, vibrant foods
Light is a frequency, not just a nutrient	Sun-charge food, eat with gratitude
Structure preserves signal	Gentle preparation and mindful storage
You are what you resonate with	Eat food that still carries the memory of the sun

The **future of nutrition** is not reductionist—it is radiant. When you eat food that still holds light, you restore your cellular memory of wholeness.

References

1. Popp FA, et al. Biophoton emission: New evidence for coherence in living biological systems. In: *Electromagnetic Bio-Information.* Urban & Schwarzenberg; 1981.

2. van Wijk R, van Wijk EPA. Biophotons and bio-communication. *J Sci Explor.* 2005;19(4):531–545.

3. Bischof M. Biophotons– The light in our cells. *J Opt Phototherapy.* 2005;13(1):2–6.

4. Popp FA, Beloussov L. *Integrative biophysics: Biophotonics.* Springer; 2003.

5. Hamblin MR. Mechanisms and applications of photobiomodulation. *AIMS Biophys.* 2017;4(3):337–361.

6. Pollack GH. *The fourth phase of water: Beyond solid, liquid, and vapor.* Ebner & Sons; 2013.

7. Fels D. Cellular communication through light. *PLoS ONE.* 2009;4(4):e5086.

8. Smith-Spangler C, et al. Are organic foods safer or healthier than conventional alternatives? *Ann Intern Med.* 2012;157(5):348–366.

9. Chaplin M. Do we underestimate the importance of water structure to cell function? *J Phys Chem B.* 2006;110(33):17387–17388.

10. Knutson MD, Leeuwenburgh C. Resveratrol and caloric restriction: The promise of sirt1 activation. *Mech Ageing Dev.* 2008;129(5):291–298.

11. Vásquez-Garibay EM, et al. Impact of cooking methods on bioactive compounds in vegetables. *Food Sci Technol Int.* 2017;23(6):532–543.

12. Popp FA. Properties of biophotons and their theoretical implications. *Indian J Exp Biol.* 2003;41(5):391–402.

13. Emoto M. *The hidden messages in water.* Atria Books; 2004.

14. Tiller WA. *Science and human transformation.* Pavior Publishing; 1997.

15. Blankenship RE, Tiede DM, Barber J, Brudvig GW, et al. Comparing photosynthetic and photovoltaic efficiencies and recognizing the potential for improvement. *Science.* 2011;332(6031):805-9.

CHAPTER 19

Quantum Meal Planning

Seasonal, Cyclical, and Individualized Strategies for Photonic Nourishment

---

Your cells don't eat just food. They eat rhythm, resonance, and relationship—with light, nature, and time.

—James Z. Liu, MD, PhD

Food as Rhythm, Not Rule

Quantum nutrition is not about rigid dietary rules; it is about aligning eating with energy, light, and biological timing. The most powerful meals are not just balanced by nutrients but by their timing, resonance, and coherence with your circadian and seasonal cycles.

This chapter explores how to design a quantum meal plan that supports physical health, biophotonic vitality, circadian alignment, and even biological age reversal by:

- Eating with the seasons of the earth
- Timing meals to the daily solar cycle
- Personalizing food choices to the biofield state
- Honoring fasting and repairing rhythms
- Building a flexible framework that evolves with you

Part I: Seasonal Eating for Photonic Synchrony

Nature feeds us on cycles. Each season encodes specific nutritional and photonic signals that harmonize with the body's needs at that time [1,2].

🌱 Spring: Cleansing and Rebirth

- Focus: Liver detox, lymphatic flow, reactivation of field coherence.
- Foods: Bitter greens (dandelion, arugula), sprouts, lemon, radish, parsley.
- Sunlight: Morning light to reset circadian rhythm post-winter.
- Practice: Raw meals, breathwork, gentle fasting.

☀️ Summer: Expansion and Energy

- Focus: Cardiovascular health, mitochondrial power, hydration.
- Foods: Raw fruits, hydrating vegetables, herbs, and cooling teas.
- Sunlight: Midday sun for vitamin D synthesis and red/NIR charging.
- Practice: Outdoor meals, grounding, structured water intake.

🍂 Autumn: Grounding and Immunity

- Focus: Lung/colon resilience, immune fortification.
- Foods: Root vegetables, cooked grains, fermented cabbage, and garlic.
- Sunlight: Afternoon sun for emotional balance.
- Practice: Warming meals, journaling, reflective practices.

❄️ Winter: Repair and Inner Light

- Focus: Kidney/adrenal restoration, melatonin balance.

- Foods: Seaweed, mushrooms, sesame, warming spices, stews.
- Sunlight: Morning light for serotonin regulation.
- Practice: Biophoton therapy, stillness, meditation.

Seasonal meals entrain your biophoton economy with Earth's electromagnetic rhythms [3,4].

Part II: Daily Photonic Timing: Eating with the Sun

Your circadian biology is a light-driven clock. Meal timing aligned with solar phases improves digestion, hormonal regulation, and mitochondrial efficiency [5,6].

Time of Day	Field Condition	Quantum Meal Strategy
Morning	Rising cortisol, low digestive fire	Light hydration: sun-charged water, fruit, enzyme-rich juice
Midday	Strongest metabolism, peak sunlight	Main photon-rich meal: raw + cooked greens, seeds, proteins
Evening	Melatonin rising, digestion waning	Warming meal: lightly cooked, fermented, calming foods
Night	Body in parasympathetic repair	Avoid food; focus on red light, breath, and coherence

Meals eaten out of sync with the sun deliver fewer photonic benefits, even if nutrients are identical [5].

Part III: Cyclical Fasting and Repair

Healing deepens in states of non-digestion. Intermittent fasting and circadian-aligned eating windows amplify autophagy, mitochondrial renewal, and photonic signaling [7,8].

Quantum-aligned fasting tips:

- Begin meals after morning sunlight exposure.
- Stop eating 2–3 hours before sleep to enhance melatonin and repair.
- Once weekly, try a 24-hour photon fast: structured water, sun, and breath only.
- Use equinoxes and solstices for 3-day raw/light detox resets.

Fasting is not deprivation; it is a recalibration of the field.

Part IV: Personalized Photonic Meal Design

Every biofield is unique. Ideal meal strategies depend on:

- Biophoton status (dim, chaotic, or coherent).
- Organ vulnerabilities (liver, gut, brain, etc.).
- Circadian type (early chronotype vs. late).
- Environment (sun-rich outdoors vs. indoor/EMF exposure).

Field Pattern	Recommended Adjustments
Low energy + brain fog	Morning structured water, red light therapy, bitter greens at lunch
Inflammation + puffiness	Sprouts, turmeric, grounding teas, and daily fermented vegetables
Anxiety + scattered focus	Root vegetables, warming cooked meals, mindful breath with food
Digestive stagnation	More raw enzymes, compressed eating window, barefoot walking

Use HRV, skin tone, sleep quality, and digestion as feedback markers to fine-tune your personal field diet [9,10].

Sample Weekly Quantum Meal Framework

Day	Photonic Focus	Meal Highlight
Monday	Liver/light detox	Dandelion greens + lemon chia water + sun walk
Tuesday	Mitochondrial charge	Beet salad + red light session + sprouted lentil bowl
Wednesday	Grounding + gut support	Kimchi broth + sweet potato + seaweed salad
Thursday	Enzyme recharge	Papaya smoothie + pranayama + sprout wrap
Friday	Cellular cleanup	Intermittent fast + structured water + early dinner
Saturday	Social grounding	Root vegetable stew + fresh herb pesto + warm cacao
Sunday	Intuitive flow	Local greens + barefoot grounding + gratitude meal prep

Summary: Eat with the Light, Live with the Light

Quantum Strategy	Nutritional Action
Align with the sun	Eat during daylight hours
Eat seasonally	Choose local, Earth-frequency foods
Build coherence through rhythm	Repeat meal cycles for stability
Customize with awareness	Adjust meals to your energy, sleep, and field feedback

Photonic nourishment is not one-size-fits-all; it is a dance with nature's cycles. When your meals honor light, time, and field, eating itself becomes a form of healing.

References

1. Lampe JW. Spicing up a vegetarian diet: chemopreventive effects of phytochemicals. *Am J Clin Nutr.* 2003;78(3 Suppl):579S–583S.

2. Van Wijk R, Van Wijk EPA. Biophoton emission and seasonal adaptation. *J Photochem Photobiol B.* 2005;79(2):141–147.

3. Popp FA et al. Biophoton emission: experimental background and theoretical approaches. *Modern Physics Letters B.* 1994;8,(21-22):1269-1296.

4. Bischof M. Biophotons–The light in our cells. *J Opt Photother.* 2005;13(1):2–6.

5. Panda S. Circadian physiology of metabolism. *Science.* 2016;354(6315):1008–1015.

6. Longo VD, Panda S. Fasting, circadian rhythms, and time-restricted feeding. *Cell Metab.* 2016;23(6):1048–1059.

7. Mattson MP, et al. Intermittent metabolic switching and cellular resilience. *N Engl J Med.* 2019;381(26):2541–2551.

8. Chaix A, et al. Time-restricted feeding is a preventative and therapeutic intervention against diverse nutritional challenges. *Cell Metab* 2014;20(6):991-1005.

9. Rubik B. The biofield hypothesis: its biophysical basis and role in medicine. *J Altern Complement Med.* 2002;8(6):703–717.

10. Shaffer F, McCraty R. Heart rate variability: a measure of autonomic coherence. *Front Public Health.* 2017;5:258.

CHAPTER 20

Integrating Biophoton Devices in Daily Life

Protocols for Energy, Sleep, and Regeneration

When light surrounds you, your body remembers how to heal.

—James Z. Liu, MD, PhD

Why Biophoton Devices Work

Healthy cells emit coherent biophotons to communicate, regulate, and repair [1,2]. In states of illness, aging, or chronic stress, this communication becomes weak, chaotic, or fragmented.

Biophoton devices provide concentrated and sustained exposure to coherent light fields, which:

- Deliver photons in the 600–950 nm range, known to stimulate mitochondrial activity [3,4].
- Recharge cytochrome c oxidase (complex IV), enhancing ATP production and cellular repair [5].
- Support immune and nervous system balance through biofield entrainment [6].
- Provide non-invasive, frequency-based regeneration, unlike chemical interventions that act only biochemically.

Key principle: Light operates as both energy and information, restoring coherence across tissues, fluids, and the biofield.

Core Types of Biophoton Devices

Device Type	Primary Frequency Range	Applications
🔴 Red/NIR Panels	600–850 nm	Mitochondrial energy, pain reduction, and collagen repair
🌀 Tesla BioHealers	Broad coherent ambient field	Sleep, regeneration, immune balance, emotional calm
💡 Biophoton-infused textiles	Passive diffusion	Sleep depth, focus, EMF field buffering
📿 Wearable light patches	Localized LED/NIR	Pain relief, targeted energy enhancement
🛏 Biophoton sleep mats	Full-body coherence field	Overnight parasympathetic repair, spinal alignment

Selection depends on lifestyle, circadian rhythm, and health goals.

Morning Protocols: Energize and Align

- Timeframe: 6:00–9:00 AM (within 30–60 minutes of sunrise)
- Goals: Activate mitochondria, sharpen mental clarity, reset circadian clock.
- Practices:
  - 10–15 minutes of red/NIR panel to face and chest.
  - Drink sun-charged or structured water.
  - Tesla BioHealer near the abdomen or liver for metabolic priming.
  - Gentle movement or breathwork (e.g., Qi Gong, sun salutations).

Red/NIR morning exposure has been shown to regulate cortisol awakening response and improve mitochondrial output [5,7].

Midday Protocols: Recharge and Digest

- Timeframe: 12:00–2:00 PM
- Goals: Support digestion, reduce inflammation, and sustain energy.
- Practices:
  - 5–10 minutes of red light over the abdomen or back.
  - Short nap with a biophoton mat or pillow.
  - Hydrate with structured water energized by sunlight or sound.

Light therapy has been shown to reduce postprandial fatigue and inflammation by enhancing nitric oxide and mitochondrial signaling [8].

Evening Protocols: Regenerate and Unwind

- Timeframe: 6:00–9:00 PM
- Goals: Reduce oxidative stress, entrain melatonin, and prepare for repair.
- Practices:
  - Tesla BioHealer near the head, chest, or feet.
  - 10 minutes of red-light panel on the spine or neck.
  - Biophoton eye masks to shield against EMF/blue-light disruption.
  - Journaling or meditation in a coherent field.

Red and infrared light in the evening helps balance circadian rhythms and improve sleep quality [9,10].

Sleep Protocols: Deep Field Repair

- Timeframe: 9:30 PM–6:00 AM
- Goals: Maximize parasympathetic repair, increase melatonin, restore mitochondrial rhythm.

- Practices:
    - Sleep near a Tesla BioHealer or on a biophoton mat.
    - Use a biophoton pillow under the spine or neck.
    - Wear biophoton-infused sleepwear or masks.
    - Add grounding sheets for Earth-field conductivity.

Expected outcomes (2–4 weeks):

- Deeper, uninterrupted sleep.
- Elevated HRV (heart rate variability).
- Morning vitality and reduced inflammation.
- Faster recovery of muscle and neural tissue.

Photobiomodulation has been shown to improve HRV, reduce sleep disturbances, and accelerate night-time mitochondrial repair [10,11].

Weekly Reset Protocol: Quantum Recharge Day

Goal: Restore coherence and clear accumulated energetic stress.

Suggested Flow:

1. Morning: Red/NIR session + raw green juice + sunrise gazing.
2. Midday: Detox bath (magnesium + structured water + Tesla device).
3. Afternoon: Restorative nap with red light near adrenals.
4. Evening: Light meal + breathwork + biophoton immersion in darkness.

Weekly photonic immersion may reset inflammatory and stress markers more effectively than daily fragmented exposure [12].

Special Use Cases

Condition	Suggested Protocol
Chronic fatigue	Morning red light + Tesla near heart + biophoton-rich food
Inflammatory pain	Local red/NIR (2x/day) + Tesla overnight field support
Brain fog/anxiety	Red light forehead + biophoton mat spine support
Detox support	Tesla near liver/kidneys + structured water
Post-exercise recovery	20 min NIR on large muscle groups + electrolyte water

Tracking the Impact

Signs of effective integration:

- Tingling/warmth during use.
- Deeper sleep, vivid dreaming.
- Lower inflammation and stiffness.
- Sharper focus and emotional stability.
- Higher HRV and improved recovery times.

Use Bio-Well scans, HRV monitoring, and sleep trackers alongside self-reflection to measure progress [6,9].

Summary: Light Belongs in Your Life

Time of Day	Device Use	Field Outcome
Morning	Red/NIR face and chest + Tesla core	Circadian reset, mitochondrial charge
Midday	Structured water + rest with biophoton mat	Detox support, field recharge
Evening	Red light spine + biophoton mask	Nervous system calm, melatonin rises
Sleep	Tesla BioHealer + grounding + dark	Parasympathetic repair, deep regeneration

Biophoton devices are not mere gadgets; they are field companions, reminding the body how to communicate, repair, and thrive in coherence.

Used consistently, they become part of a light-based lifestyle: one that nourishes not just your cells but the luminous blueprint of life itself.

References

1. Popp FA, Gu Q, Li KH. Biophoton emission: experimental background and theoretical approaches. *Mod Phys Lett B.* 1994;8(21-22):1269-1296.

2. van Wijk R, van Wijk EPA. Biophoton communication and regulation in living systems. *J Photochem Photobiol B.* 2005;79(2):141–147.

3. Hamblin MR. Mechanisms and applications of the anti-inflammatory effects of photobiomodulation. *AIMS Biophysics.* 2017;4(3):337–361.

4. Chung H, et al. The nuts and bolts of low-level laser (light) therapy. *Ann Biomed Eng.* 2012;40(2):516–533.

5. Karu TI. Mitochondrial mechanisms of photobiomodulation in context of new data about multiple roles of ATP. *Photomed Laser Surg.* 2010;28(2):159–160.

6. Rubik B. The biofield hypothesis: its biophysical basis and role in medicine. *J Altern Complement Med.* 2002;8(6):703–717.

7. LeGates TA, Fernandez DC, Hattar S. Light as a central modulator of circadian rhythms, sleep, and affect. *Nat Rev Neurosci.* 2014;15(7):443–454.

8. Passarella S, Karu T. Absorption of monochromatic and narrow band radiation in the visible and near IR by cytochrome c oxidase. *J Photochem Photobiol B.* 2014;140:344–358.

9. Tonello L, et al. Photobiomodulation therapy for sleep disorders: A systematic review. *Sleep Med.* 2021;80:203–211.

10. Schiffer F, et al. Psychological benefits of near-infrared light to the brain. *Behav Brain Funct.* 2009;5:46.

11. Rentz LE, Bryner RW, Ramadan J, Rezai A, Galster SM. Full-body photobiomodulation therapy is associated with reduced sleep durations and augmented cardiorespiratory indicators of recovery. *Sports (Basel).* 2022;10(8):119.

12. Salehpour F, et al. Transcranial photobiomodulation therapy: a narrative review. *Rev Neurosci.* 2018;29(5):427–441.

CHAPTER 21

Quantum Nutrition for Pets

Extending Vibrational Health Beyond Humans

Biophotons do not recognize species. Where there is life, there is light. Where there is light, there is the potential for healing.

—James Z. Liu, MD, PhD

The Universal Language of Light in Animals

Quantum nutrition extends beyond human biology. Just as people rely on coherent light for cellular communication, pets—dogs, cats, horses, and other animals—also emit and absorb ultra-weak photon emissions (biophotons) from their DNA and mitochondria. These emissions serve as a direct indicator of vitality and order in living systems [1,2].

Pets, often even more sensitive than humans, naturally seek out sources of coherent energy: lying in sunlit spaces, grounding themselves on the earth, or curling up near biophoton devices. Recognizing and supporting this innate connection to light helps reverse age-related decline, improve mobility, and restore emotional balance in animals.

Biophoton Basics for Pets

Just like humans, companion animals:

- Emit and absorb photons as part of normal physiology [1].

- Depend on mitochondrial ATP and structured water for energy balance [3].
- Respond strongly to red and near-infrared (NIR) light, which supports tissue healing and circulation [4,6].
- Exhibit measurable changes in physiology when exposed to coherent fields [5].

Signs of "Low-Field" Health in Pets:

- Lethargy or restlessness.
- Dull or patchy coat, skin irritation.
- Sluggish digestion or irregular elimination.
- Joint stiffness or reduced mobility.
- Anxiety, agitation, or disrupted sleep.

Key Insight: Many pets instinctively seek out coherence. Their attraction to sunny spots or calm energy fields is evidence of their innate sensitivity to vibrational order.

Quantum Inputs for Pet Wellness

Input	Application	Expected Benefit
Tesla BioHealer (Pet Size)	Place near the pet's bed or crate	Stem cell activation, joint repair, and calmness
Red/NIR Light Therapy	5–10 min on hips, spine, or injury site	Mobility, circulation, tissue repair [4,6]
Structured Water	Daily drinking source with minerals	Hydration, detox, mitochondrial support [3]
Raw/Vibrational Foods	Add small amounts of greens/fermented veggies	Gut microbiome balance, coat health [7]
Natural Light Exposure	Morning outdoor time	Circadian entrainment, hormonal balance [8]

Case Snapshot: Restoring Vitality in a Dog

A nine-year-old Labrador with chronic stiffness, fatigue, and digestive issues was introduced to two interventions:

1. Structured water enriched with chlorophyll.
2. Nighttime exposure to a Tesla BioHealer near its sleeping area.

Outcomes within 10 days:

- Energy levels increased.
- Mobility improved noticeably.
- Digestion normalized.
- Skin irritation resolved.

Veterinary observation suggested that coherence in the biofield and mitochondrial balance was restored without the need for pharmacological intervention.

Harmonizing the Home Field with Pets

When pets receive biophoton nourishment alongside their human companions, the household itself becomes a regenerative ecosystem. A coherent home field benefits both animals and people through shared vibrational stability.

Practical Suggestions for Pet-Integrated Coherence:

- Place a central biophoton device in common living areas.
- Allow pets to share red light or BioHealer sessions.
- Pair outdoor walks with sunlight and grounding for both the owner and the animal.
- Integrate structured water bowls to ensure hydration coherence.

This is not just pet care, it is field care, cultivating resonance across species within the same household.

Summary: Pets Thrive in Light

Being	Biophoton Benefit	Simple Action
🐶 Pets	Vitality, mobility, emotional calm	Add Tesla BioHealer sessions + red/NIR light therapy
🏠 Home	Harmonized energetic atmosphere	Central device + shared coherence practices

Quantum nutrition is not isolated to humans. By extending coherent light to companion animals, you support their vitality, longevity, and emotional well-being. Pets flourish when their environment nourishes their light, creating a mutually healing field that benefits all members of the household.

References

1. Popp FA, Gu Q, Li KH. Biophoton emission: experimental background and theoretical approaches. *Mod Phys Lett B.* 1994;8(21-22):1269-1296.

2. Van Wijk R, Van Wijk EPA. An introduction to human biophoton emission. *Forsch Komplementarmed Klass Naturheilkd.* 2005;12(2):77-83.

3. Pollack GH. *The fourth phase of water.* Ebner & Sons; 2013.

4. Chung H, et al. The nuts and bolts of low-level laser (light) therapy. *Ann Biomed Eng.* 2012;40(2):516–533.

5. Rubik B. The biofield hypothesis: its biophysical basis and role in medicine. *J Altern Complement Med.* 2002;8(6):703–717.

6. Hamblin MR. Photobiomodulation for animals: Evidence and mechanisms. *Vet Sci.* 2020;7(4):188.

7. Swanson KS, et al. Nutrition and the microbiome in companion animals. *Front Microbiol.* 2021;12:651110.

8. LeGates TA, Fernandez DC, Hattar S. Light as a central modulator of circadian rhythms, sleep, and affect. *Nat Rev Neurosci.* 2014;15(7):443–454.

CHAPTER 22

Quantum Nutrition for Plants

Extending Healthy Food Supply

Plants are the Earth's original solar panels. To nourish them with coherent light is to amplify the foundation of all life.

—James Z. Liu, MD, PhD

The Plant–Photon Connection

Plants are natural light antennas. Through photosynthesis, they capture photons from the sun and convert them into chemical energy, which sustains not only their growth but also the entire food web. Beyond photosynthesis, plants also emit ultra-weak photon emissions (biophotons) from their DNA, mitochondria, and chloroplasts [1,2]. These emissions serve as indicators of plant vitality, coherence, and stress resistance.

Modern agriculture often prioritizes yield through chemical inputs, while neglecting the energetic integrity of plants. This leads to produce that may be abundant in quantity but diminished in vibrational quality—foods with lower levels of antioxidants, enzymes, and photonic coherence [3,4]. Quantum nutrition for plants shifts the focus from material inputs (fertilizers, pesticides) to light-based nourishment that restores vitality and sustainability.

Signs of Low-Photon Plants

- Faster wilting or poor shelf-life.
- Dull coloration, reduced chlorophyll density.
- Lower resistance to pests, mold, and drought.
- Decreased nutrient and antioxidant content.
- Weak or inconsistent growth patterns.

Key Insight: A plant's photon field is directly tied to its nutritional and medicinal value. High-biophoton plants not only thrive longer but also nourish humans and animals with greater coherence.

Quantum Inputs for Plant Health

Input	**Application**	**Expected Benefit**
🌞 Natural Sunlight Rhythms	Morning and full-spectrum exposure	Synchronizes photosynthesis, boosts coherence [5]
💧 Structured Water Irrigation	Charged with sunlight or biophoton field	Improves hydration, enzymatic activity [6]
🌀 Biophoton Generators	Placed near crops or greenhouses	Enhances germination, growth rate [7]
🥦 Sprouting in Coherent Fields	Indoor trays under structured conditions	Highest photon-emitting microgreens [8]
🎶 Sound and Intention	Classical music, 432 Hz, mindful care	Improves growth and field organization [9]

Scientific Insights

- Chlorophyll stability: Biophoton-enhanced plants show delayed chlorophyll degradation, preserving greener leaves and higher photosynthetic efficiency [5,10].

- Stronger root systems: Photon stimulation promotes deeper, thicker roots, supporting nutrient absorption and drought resilience [7].
- Antioxidant production: Enhanced synthesis of polyphenols and vitamins boosts both plant survival and human nutrition [11].
- Pest and disease resistance: Light-based coherence reduces susceptibility to fungal and bacterial infections [12].
- Shelf-life extension: Fresh produce exposed to biophoton fields retains its firmness, aroma, and nutrient content for a longer period post-harvest [13].

Applications Across Plant Systems

- Home gardens: Adding structured water and small biophoton devices improves the flavor, vitality, and resilience of herbs and vegetables.
- Commercial farming: Integrating photonic technologies reduces dependence on pesticides and fertilizers, cutting costs while enhancing yields.
- Greenhouses and vertical farms: Coherent light fields support controlled-environment agriculture, boosting efficiency and sustainability.
- Post-harvest storage: Biophoton exposure extends freshness, reducing waste along supply chains.

Case Snapshot: Lettuce in Biophoton Fields

In controlled greenhouse trials, lettuce grown near biophoton generators demonstrated:

- 25–30% faster growth rate.
- Higher chlorophyll density produces richer color and taste.

- Longer post-harvest freshness, with reduced wilting after one week in storage.
  These results align with earlier studies, which show that plants exposed to coherent light develop stronger electromagnetic order and resilience [7,12].

Toward a Photonic Agriculture

The future of farming may shift from chemical reliance to light-based cultivation:

- Farmers using biophoton devices report healthier soils and crops with greater vitality.
- Organic agriculture benefits by reducing the need for chemical preservatives and pesticides.
- Communities gain fresher, more nutrient-dense produce with longer shelf life.

Quantum nutrition in agriculture supports not just crop yields, but the entire food supply chain, from soil vitality to consumer health.

Summary: Plants as Carriers of Light

Domain	Quantum Benefit	Practical Action
🌱 Plants	Higher vitality, resistance, yield	Use structured water + biophoton fields
🍎 Produce	Fresher, nutrient-rich food	Post-harvest biophoton preservation
🌍 Agriculture	Sustainable, chemical-free farming	Integrate photonic technologies in fields

By nourishing plants with biophotons, we strengthen the foundation of global food security. When fruits, vegetables, and grains store and transmit coherent light, they not only feed human bodies but also elevate the vibrational health of societies and ecosystems.

References

1. Popp FA, Gu Q, Li KH. Biophoton emission: experimental background and theoretical approaches. *Mod Phys Lett B.* 1994;8(21-22):1269-1296.

2. Van Wijk R, Van Wijk EPA. An introduction to human biophoton emission. *Forsch Komplementarmed Klass Naturheilkd.* 2005;12(2):77-83.

3. Foley JA, et al. Solutions for a cultivated planet. *Nature.* 2011;478(7369):337–342.

4. Altmann H. Sustainable agriculture and the role of innovative biotechnologies. *Agric Syst.* 2014;123:9–20.

5. Nassarawa SS, Abdullah Sani N, Zawawi N, Ding P. Effect of light-emitting diodes (LEDs) on the quality of fruits and vegetables during postharvest period: A review. *Food Bioprocess Technol.* 2021;14(1):1-27.

6. Pollack GH. *The fourth phase of water.* Ebner & Sons; 2013.

7. Mould RR et al. Ultra weak photon emission—a brief review. *Front Physiol.* 2024 Feb 14;15:1348915.

8. Bischof M. *Biophotons—The light in our cells.* Integrative Biophysics. Springer; 2008.

9. Liu Z, Fadiji T, Yang J, Li Z, Tchuenbou-Magaia F. Impact of mechanical stimulation on the life cycle of horticultural plant. *Horticultural Plant Journal.* 2023;9(3):381-394.

10. Yamauchi N, Watada AE. Chlorophyll and xanthophyll changes in broccoli florets stored under elevated CO_2 and/or reduced O_2. *Postharvest Biol Technol.* 1991;1(2):109–116.

11. Mittler R. Oxidative stress, antioxidants, and stress tolerance in plants. *Trends Plant Sci.* 2002;7(9):405–410.

12. Musumeci F, et al. Coherence and electromagnetic order in plant development. *Bioelectromagnetics.* 2011;32(6):420–430.

13. Prasad A. et al. Spectral distribution of ultra-weak photon emission as a response to wounding in plants: An in vivo study. *Biology (Basel).* 2020 Jun 26;9(6):139. doi: 10.3390/biology9060139.

CHAPTER 23

Quantum Nutrition in Medicine and Longevity

Applications in Chronic Disease and Age Reversal

Medicine that heals must speak the language of light.
Only then can we reverse the entropy of aging.
—James Z. Liu, MD, PhD

Quantum Nutrition as Medicine

Quantum nutrition is more than a personal wellness path. It is the emerging foundation of a new medical paradigm—one that addresses chronic disease, extends healthspan, and targets biological aging at its informational and energetic roots.

Biophoton-centered care is beginning to integrate into:

- Preventive and integrative medicine
- Chronic disease management and reversal
- Longevity and regenerative therapies
- Hospital and rehabilitation protocols
- Personalized, AI-assisted care

At its heart is a profound insight: aging and disease are not inevitable declines but reversible disorders of coherence and light [1,2]. When the body's field is re-ordered through quantum inputs—light, water, food, frequency, and intention—cells often remember how to regenerate.

Quantum Aging: The Biology of Disintegration

Classical science measures aging by:

- Mitochondrial decline and reduced ATP output [3].
- Telomere shortening with each cell division [4].
- Epigenetic drift disrupting gene regulation [5].
- Protein glycation and misfolding, stiffening tissues [6].
- Stem cell exhaustion, reducing repair capacity [7].

Quantum biology provides a deeper insight: aging is also characterized by the progressive loss of electromagnetic coherence and biofield integrity [8,9].

When coherence is lost:

- Mitochondria emit less biophotonic light.
- DNA repair enzymes misfire.
- Tissues lose electrical charge and hydration [10].
- Cells enter senescence instead of renewal.

This is entropy in action—light lost, structure scrambled, renewal silenced.

Biophotonic Interventions: A New Class of Therapy

Quantum nutrition introduces **non-invasive interventions** that reverse aging by recharging, realigning, and restoring biological order.

Quantum Tool	Anti-Aging Mechanism
● Red/NIR Light (600–900 nm)	Stimulates cytochrome c oxidase, boosts ATP, supports collagen and stem cells [11,12]
Tesla BioHealer	Provides coherent field exposure; may enhance stem cell signaling, deep recovery [13]

Quantum Tool	Anti-Aging Mechanism
Structured Water	Restores intracellular hydration, improves protein folding [10,14]
Raw Biophoton Foods	Supply antioxidants, enzymes, and coherent photon emissions [2,15]
Circadian Sunlight	Regulates melatonin, serotonin, and mitochondrial rhythms [16]

Together, these inputs target the root drivers of aging: mitochondrial stagnation, inflammation, glycation, and loss of field order.

Clinical Applications: Quantum Nutrition in Chronic Disease

Neurodegenerative Disorders (Alzheimer's, Parkinson's)

- Photobiomodulation (red/NIR therapy) to the skull/scalp improves memory and cognition [17].
- Tesla field devices may stabilize sleep and reduce tremors.
- Biophoton-rich ketogenic diets reduce neuroinflammation [18].
- Circadian light entrainment enhances mood and circadian regulation [16].

Patients report sharper memory, steadier gait, and improved emotional presence.

Cardiovascular Disease

- Biophoton-rich diets reduce oxidative stress and inflammation [15].
- Red/NIR light enhances vascular dilation by releasing nitric oxide [19].

- Structured water improves red blood cell flexibility, enhancing perfusion [10].
- *Improved blood pressure and reduced medication needs within weeks.*

Cancer and Immune Disorders

- Biophotons enhance mitochondrial signaling and immune surveillance [20].
- Structured water and coherent foods reduce tumor-promoting inflammation [14,15].
- Photonic therapies reduce fatigue during chemotherapy [21].
- *Not a cure, but a field-strengthening adjunct improving outcomes and quality of life.*

Chronic Pain and Inflammation

- Red/NIR light reduces nerve pain and joint inflammation [22].
- Tesla BioHealers support pain reduction without drugs [13].
- Breathwork + field therapy enhances vagal tone and endorphin cycles [8].
- *Quantum pain protocols often yield a 50–80% reduction in symptoms within 1–3 weeks.*

Quantum Longevity Protocols

Aging can now be measured, tracked, and reversed. Longevity clinics integrate biophoton strategies with biometrics:

Metric	Quantum Optimization
Epigenetic Age	Improved through red/NIR light, fasting, raw plant nutrients [5,11]

Metric	Quantum Optimization
HRV (Heart Rate Variability)	Guided with breathwork, biophoton devices, coherence training [8,9]
GDV/Biofield Imaging	Detects systemic coherence shifts after quantum inputs [9,23]
Telomere Length	Supported via reduced oxidative stress and improved mitochondrial function [4,19]
Sleep Architecture	Enhanced by circadian sunlight and field-assisted sleep [16]

Some clinics combine AI, biofield imaging, light prescriptions, and EMF-free environments to extend vitality by decades.

Hospitals and Rehabilitation Centers

Forward-thinking hospitals are piloting:

- Red/NIR light beds for surgical recovery [21].
- Biophoton devices in neurology wings for neuro-rehab.
- Enzyme-preserved, raw meal programs in oncology wards.
- Field-enhancing textiles to reduce patient stress.

Reported outcomes: faster wound healing, less anxiety, lower medication use.

Toward Quantum Primary Care

Imagine your annual check-up including:

- A biofield scan to detect disharmony before disease.
- AI-analyzed light maps of organs and tissues.
- A personalized red light + food prescription for your field state.

- Guidance on photonic supplementation, grounding, and breath cycles.

This is medicine that works in resonance with life's intelligence; health measured in watts, not just words.

Summary: Quantum Nutrition as a Medical Revolution

Target	Quantum Approach
Aging	Restore field coherence, re-energize mitochondria
Chronic disease	Reduce inflammation, glycation, and incoherence
Regeneration	Activate stem cells with coherent inputs
Longevity	Track biological age with photonic and energetic markers
Medicine	Shift from suppression → illumination

Light heals where drugs cannot.
Structure restores what surgery removes.
Field coherence awakens what time erodes.

Quantum nutrition is not fringe; it is the seed of a medical revolution, honoring biology as a frequency network and life as a symphony of light.

References

1. Popp FA et al. Biophoton emission: experimental background and theoretical approaches. *Modern Physics Letters B.* 1994;8(21-22):1269–1296.

2. van Wijk R, van Wijk EPA. Biophoton communication and regulation in living systems. *J Photochem Photobiol B.* 2005;79(2):141–147.

3. Sun N, Youle RJ, Finkel T. The mitochondrial basis of aging. *Mol Cell.* 2016;61(5):654-666. doi:10.1016/j.molcel.2016.01.028.

4. Blackburn EH, Epel ES. Telomeres and adversity: Too toxic to ignore. *Nature.* 2012;490(7419):169-171. doi:10.1038/490169a.
(Note: there is no widely indexed "Telomeres and aging" article in Annu Rev Psychol in 2012 under these authors.)

5. Horvath S, Raj K. DNA methylation-based biomarkers and the epigenetic clock theory of ageing. *Nat Rev Genet.* 2018;19(6):371-384. doi:10.1038/s41576-018-0004-3.

6. Brownlee M. The pathobiology of diabetic complications: A unifying mechanism. *Diabetes.* 2005;54(6):1615-1625. doi:10.2337/diabetes.54.6.1615.

7. López-Otín C, Blasco MA, Partridge L, Serrano M, Kroemer G. The hallmarks of aging. *Cell.* 2013;153(6):1194-1217.

8. Biofield Rubik B. The biofield hypothesis: Its biophysical basis and role in medicine. *J Altern Complement Med.* 2002;8(6):703-717.

9. Korotkov KG. *Human Energy Field: Study with GDV Bioelectrography.* Fair Lawn, NJ: Backbone Publishing Co.; 2002.

10. Pollack GH. *The Fourth Phase of Water: Beyond Solid, Liquid, and Vapor.* Seattle, WA: Ebner & Sons Publishers; 2013.

11. Hamblin MR. Mechanisms and applications of the anti-inflammatory effects of photobiomodulation. In: *Proc SPIE.* 2018;10477:104770T.

12. Chung H, Dai T, Sharma SK, Huang YY, Carroll JD, Hamblin MR. The nuts and bolts of low-level laser (light) therapy. *Ann Biomed Eng.* 2012;40(2):516-533.

13. Liu JZ, Smotrys MA, Robinson SD, Yu HX, Liu SX, Liu DR, and Gu HY. Title: Biophoton Therapy for Chronic Pain: Clinical and Real-World Breakthrough. J Neurol Res Rev Rep, 2025 Volume 7(7): 46-54.

14. Chai B, Yoo H, Pollack GH. Effect of radiant energy on near-surface water. *J Phys Chem B.* 2009;113(42):13953-13958.

15. Bischof M. *Biophotons: The Light in Our Cells.* Frankfurt, Germany: Zweitausendeins; 2008.

16. LeGates TA, Fernandez DC, Hattar S. Light as a central modulator of circadian rhythms, sleep and affect. *Nat Rev Neurosci.* 2014;15(7):443-454. doi:10.1038/nrn3743.

17. Saltmarche AE, Naeser MA, Ho KF, Hamblin MR, Lim L. Significant improvement in cognitive performance post-transcranial, intranasal, and intrafocal photobiomodulation therapy in a patient with dementia. *Photomed Laser Surg.* 2017;35(10):605-610.

18. Bredesen DE. Reversal of cognitive decline: A novel therapeutic program. *Aging (Albany NY).* 2014;6(9):707-717.

19. Mitchell UH, Mack GL. Low-level laser treatment for ankle sprains and chronic pain: A review of mechanisms involving nitric oxide. *Lasers Surg Med.* 2013;45(1):1-10.

20. Whelan HT, Smits RL Jr, Buchmann EV, et al. Effect of NASA light-emitting diode irradiation on wound healing. *J Clin Laser Med Surg.* 2001;19(6):305-314.

21. Salehpour F, Mahmoudi J, Kamari F, Sadigh-Eteghad S, Rasta SH, Hamblin MR. Brain photobiomodulation therapy: A narrative review. *Mol Neurobiol.* 2018;55(8):6601-6636.

22. de Freitas LF, Hamblin MR. Proposed mechanisms of photobiomodulation or low-level light therapy. *IEEE J Sel Top Quantum Electron.* 2016;22(3):7000417.

23. Fels D. Cellular communication through light. *PLoS ONE.* 2009;4(4):e5086.

CHAPTER 24

AI, Frequency Mapping, and Personalized Nutrition

Merging Technology with Biofield Science for the Future of Wellness

---

When AI learns to read our frequencies, nutrition becomes a dialogue between intelligence and resonance.

—James Z. Liu, MD, PhD

From Food Pyramids to Frequency Maps

Traditional nutrition has long relied on static models, such as calories, macronutrients, and food pyramids, that assume a universal template for all humans. However, research now shows that individual biological rhythms, circadian cycles, and energetic states dramatically influence nutritional needs [1,2].

Quantum nutrition reframes food as information encoded in light and vibration. Since each person has a unique electromagnetic and biophotonic signature, nutritional strategies should adapt dynamically to:

- Circadian timing and sunlight exposure [3].
- Stress, sleep, and emotional states [4].
- Environmental fields (EMF, grounding, geophysical rhythms) [5].

Frequency mapping makes these invisible dynamics visible, while Artificial Intelligence (AI) interprets patterns too subtle for the human mind alone.

What Is Frequency Mapping?

Frequency mapping refers to the measurement and visualization of oscillatory patterns within the human biofield. These patterns include:

- Biophoton emissions from tissues and organs [6,7].
- Electromagnetic coherence, measured through HRV, EEG, or voltage gradients [8].
- Resonant signatures of chakras and meridians, observed in GDV/Bio-Well imaging [9].
- Bioelectrical impedance and membrane potential shifts [10].

Using tools like Gas Discharge Visualization (GDV), EEG/HRV devices, voice frequency analysis, and near-infrared imaging, clinicians can now generate a real-time map of vibrational health. These scans highlight areas of coherence, deficiency, or blockage before physical disease manifests [8,9].

Enter AI: Translating Frequencies into Nutrition

AI acts as a **translator** between frequency data and actionable interventions. Machine learning systems can:

AI Function	**Application in Quantum Nutrition**
📊 Analyze coherence/entropy trends	Detect subtle imbalances or "aging hotspots" before symptoms appear [11]
🧠 Predict energetic needs	Suggest light-based therapies, coherence foods, or detox strategies [12]
🍽 Dynamic meal design	Adjust meal composition and timing in real time via HRV/field scans [13]
🔴 Adaptive light/EMF modulation	Tune red/NIR light or block EMF according to circadian and mitochondrial state

AI Function	Application in Quantum Nutrition
🧬 Genetic + frequency integration	Combine epigenetic clocks with vibrational data for deeper personalization [14]

AI doesn't replace human intuition. Instead, it augments it, allowing nutrition to become a conversation between the body's field and intelligence systems.

A Day in the Life: AI-Driven Quantum Nutrition (2035)

- Morning scan: Your wearable collects HRV, EEG, and mitochondrial data during sleep.
- AI assistant (QuantumCareTM) notes:
  "Liver field shows mild congestion. Solar plexus coherence is low. EMF overload from yesterday's travel detected."
- Recommendations:
  - Warm lemon–dandelion infusion for detox.
  - Red light therapy on the lower back (10 minutes).
  - A 6-hour eating window with sprouted greens and fermented vegetables.
  - A guided breath session paired with 432 Hz tones.

Nutrition, light, water, and breath are now dynamically aligned with your real-time biofield.

Emerging Technologies

Technology	Quantum Nutrition Role
🧬 Epigenetic + Biophoton Integration	Cross-reference DNA methylation age with live photon emissions [14,15]

Technology	Quantum Nutrition Role
🤖 AI-Powered Biofield Analysis	Interpret HRV, voice tone, or GDV scans for coherence tracking [11,13]
⚫ Adaptive Photonic Wearables	Deliver red/NIR light where needed, tuned in real time [16]
📱 Quantum Nutrition Apps	Provide daily food and light schedules based on field scans
🧠 Brain–Gut–Field Feedback	Connect emotional state to gut health and photonic needs [17]

These technologies are not about control, but about **revealing nature's intelligence** and making it actionable.

Human + AI: A Coherent Partnership

In quantum medicine, AI is not a replacement for intuition but a partner in coherence.

- It helps us see what the body already feels but cannot verbalize.
- It recognizes patterns across millions of data points that humans miss.
- It adapts more quickly to stress, travel, and aging shifts.
- It frees space for heart-centered healing and consciousness practices.

The future healer is hybrid: Soul + Sensor, Intuition + Intelligence, Nature + Network.

Ethical Boundaries

As with all powerful tools, ethics must guide development:

- Consent and privacy in biofield scans [18].

- AI should empower self-healing, not medical dependency.
- Data must remain encrypted and sovereign.
- The biofield should be honored as sacred, not reduced to code.

Quantum nutrition must remain a path to sovereignty, not surveillance.

Summary: From Biofeedback to Biofrequency

Traditional Approach	Quantum–AI Approach
Static diet templates	Adaptive meals tuned to frequency states
Reliance on blood labs and symptoms	Real-time biofield + mitochondrial diagnostics
Generalized supplementation	Personalized photon-rich foods and light prescriptions
Reactive treatments	Proactive coherence optimization

With AI and frequency mapping, nutrition becomes a living dialogue between your body and its environment. You are no longer guessing—you are listening to your own light.

What emerges is not just better health, but a new relationship with the body as a conscious field of intelligence and resonance.

References

1. van Ommen B, van der Greef J, Ordovas JM, Daniel H. Phenotypic flexibility as key factor in the human nutrition and health relationship. *Nat Rev Gastroenterol Hepatol.* 2014;11(11):631-636. doi:10.1038/nrgastro.2014.98.

2. Zee PC, Attarian H, Videnovic A. Circadian rhythm abnormalities. *Continuum (Minneap Minn).* 2013;19(1 Sleep Disorders):132-147.

3. LeGates TA, Fernandez DC, Hattar S. Light as a central modulator of circadian rhythms, sleep and affect. *Nat Rev Neurosci.* 2014;15(7):443-454. doi:10.1038/nrn3743.

4. McEwen BS. Protective and damaging effects of stress mediators. *N Engl J Med.* 1998;338(3):171-179. doi:10.1056/NEJM199801153380307.

5. Magnetic Field Buchachenko AL, Kouznetsov DA, Arkhangelsky SE, Orlova MA, Markarian AA. Magnetic isotope effect in biology and medicine. *Bioelectromagnetics.* 2017;38(1):1-12. doi:10.1002/bem.22015.

6. Popp FA, Gu Q, Li KH. Biophoton emission: Experimental background and theoretical approaches. *Mod Phys Lett B.* 1994;8(21-22):1269-1296. doi:10.1142/S0217984994001266.

7. van Wijk R, van Wijk EPA. Multi-site recording and spectral analysis of spontaneous photon emission from human body. *Forsch Komplementmed.* 2005;12(2):96-106. doi:10.1159/000083766.

8. Shaffer F, Ginsberg JP. An overview of heart rate variability metrics and norms. *Front Public Health.* 2017;5:258. doi:10.3389/fpubh.2017.00258.

9. Korotkov KG. *Human Energy Field: Study with GDV Bioelectrography.* Fair Lawn, NJ: Backbone Publishing Co.; 2002.

10. Honigmann A, van den Bogaart G, Iraheta E, et al. A lipid bound actin meshwork organizes liquid phase separation in model membranes. *eLife*. 2014;3:e01671

11. Esteva A, Robicquet A, Ramsundar B, et al. A guide to deep learning in healthcare. *Nat Med.* 2019;25(1):24-29. doi:10.1038/s41591-018-0316-z.

12. Topol EJ. High-performance medicine: The convergence of human and artificial intelligence. *Nat Med.* 2019;25(1):44-56. doi:10.1038/s41591-018-0300-7.

13. D'Alfonso S, O'Connor A, Kyrou I, Randeva HS. Artificial intelligence and machine learning in personalized nutrition: Current applications, challenges, and future perspectives. *Nutrients.* 2023;15(6):1458. doi:10.3390/nu15061458.

14. Horvath S, Raj K. DNA methylation-based biomarkers and the epigenetic clock theory of ageing. *Nat Rev Genet.* 2018;19(6):371-384. doi:10.1038/s41576-018-0004-3.

15. Fels D. Cellular communication through light. *PLoS One.* 2009;4(4):e5086. doi:10.1371/journal.pone.0005086.

16. Hamblin MR. Mechanisms and applications of the anti-inflammatory effects of photobiomodulation. *AIMS Biophys.* 2017;4(3):337-361.

17. Mayer EA. Gut feelings: The emerging biology of gut-brain communication. *Nat Rev Neurosci.* 2011;12(8):453-466.

18. Mittelstadt BD. Principles alone cannot guarantee ethical AI. *Nat Med.* 2019;25(1):44-48.

CHAPTER 25

Rewriting the Human Health Paradigm

How Quantum Nutrition Can Transform Global Wellness

When we feed the light in each cell, we rewrite not only biology, but the future of medicine, agriculture, and the soul of society. —**James Z. Liu, MD, PhD**

The Crisis: A System That Forgot the Field

Modern health systems remain locked in mechanistic reductionism:

- Cells are viewed as isolated machines.
- Food has been reduced to calories and macronutrients.
- Illness is treated through suppression rather than regeneration.
- Aging is accepted as an inevitable decline.

This fragmented paradigm has produced:

- A global metabolic epidemic—obesity, diabetes, and chronic inflammation [1].
- Rising neurodegenerative and cardiovascular disease [2].
- Escalating mental health crises [3].
- Agricultural soil depletion and declining food quality [4].
- Widespread emotional and spiritual disconnection.

We forgot a fundamental truth: life is not only biochemical—it is bioelectromagnetic. Healing must therefore begin by restoring coherence and light within biological systems [5,6].

The Solution: A Quantum Model of Wellness

Quantum nutrition reframes wellness by addressing the **energetic distortions** underlying global health challenges.

Distortion	Quantum Correction
Nutritional depletion	Raw, enzyme-rich, biophoton-dense foods [7].
Mitochondrial decay	Recharge with red/NIR light, structured water, and grounding [8,9].
Chronic inflammation and glycation	Correct via fasting, biophoton therapies, and detoxification [10].
Circadian and seasonal disconnection	Re-align with natural light cycles, seasonal eating, and Earth-based living [11].
Fragmented healing disciplines	Integrate food, frequency, emotion, and environment into unified care [12].

This approach does not compete with modern medicine; it expands it. The human organism is not just a machine but a self-regulating field of intelligent energy [6].

A New Healthcare Blueprint: Light First, Drugs Last

Envision a global wellness model where:

- Children learn breathing, grounding, and sprout-growing in schools.
- Hospitals integrate phototherapy, structured water, and biofield monitoring alongside conventional care.
- Homes include a biophoton wellness corner with light and coherence tools.

- Physicians are trained in field diagnostics and frequency-based repair.
- Elders access technologies to reverse biological age and maintain vitality.

Medicine evolves from:

- Treat → Illuminate
- Fight → Harmonize
- Survive → Regenerate

This is not utopia; it is the natural direction of a photonic biology paradigm [5,8,13].

Education: Teaching Light Before Labels

To embed quantum nutrition, education must change first. Future curricula should be integrated:

- The role of biophotons in health and cellular communication [6,7].
- The science of structured water and electromagnetic biology [9].
- The physiology of coherence and emotional frequency [14].
- The living intelligence of food beyond macros [7,15].
- The ethics of AI and frequency diagnostics in medicine [16].

By teaching that thoughts carry frequency, food carries light, and breath carries rhythm, we equip future generations to heal through awareness, not avoidance.

Agriculture and Food Systems: A Photonic Revolution

Global wellness cannot thrive on dead soil and denatured food. Agriculture must evolve toward light-based vitality systems.

Conventional Agriculture	Quantum Agriculture
Yield and profit focus	Vitality and coherence focus
Heavy pesticides and GMOs	Regenerative, biodynamic practices
Long-distance transport	Local photonic food loops
Energy ignored	Structured water, solar-informed harvesting

Biophoton-rich crops are:

- More resilient to disease [17].
- Higher in nutrient density [18].
- Longer shelf life due to coherent structure [19].
- More healing for people, pets, and ecosystems alike.

Restoring light to soil and food is the most direct way to restore human vitality [7].

Quantum Equity: Making Light Accessible

Biophotonic nutrition and therapies must not become elite luxuries. Instead, they must be:

- Democratized through community education and empowerment.
- Scaled with open-source photonic and water-structuring technologies.

- Embedded in schools, clinics, and public wellness centers.
- Recognized by health systems as cost-saving and preventive [20].

It is not merely healthcare policy; it is vibrational justice.

Case Snapshot: A Community Reverses Its Health Crisis

In a mid-sized town facing rising obesity and type 2 diabetes, a wellness initiative introduced:

- Tesla BioHealers in senior homes and community clinics.
- Biophoton food workshops to teach sprouting, fermentation, and raw nutrition.
- Structured water stations installed in schools.
- A public sunlight meditation garden to encourage circadian alignment.

Within six months:

- 38% reduction in blood pressure medication use.
- Twofold improvement in self-reported sleep quality.
- Higher classroom focus and fewer behavioral outbursts.
- Stronger sense of community, calm, and connection.

When one field is restored, many lives are transformed.

Summary: The Path Forward Is Lit from Within

Old Paradigm	Quantum Paradigm
Disease management	Field restoration and light renewal
Food as fuel	Food as light, information, and coherence

Doctors as fixers	Humans are self-healing beings guided by frequency
Aging as an inevitable decline	Aging as a reversible loss of coherence and structure
Healthcare for symptoms	Quantum care for systems, spirit, and regeneration

We now know how to:

- Restore the Earth's light in our food.
- Restore the body's coherence through photonic nutrition.
- Restore the mind through resonance and frequency.

Quantum nutrition is not just science; it is a movement.
It is the return to truth: every living being is light in form, and nourishing that light is how we rewrite the future of human health—globally, equitably, and sustainably.

References

1. World Health Organization World Health Organization. *Global Report on Diabetes.* Geneva, Switzerland: World Health Organization; 2016.

2. Neurodegenerative Disease Hou Y, Dan X, Babbar M, et al. Ageing as a risk factor for neurodegenerative disease. *Nat Rev Neurol.* 2019;15(10):565-581.

3. Mental Illness Vigo D, Thornicroft G, Atun R. Estimating the true global burden of mental illness. *Lancet Psychiatry.* 2016;3(2):171-178.

4. Soil Health Lal R. Soil health and carbon management. *Food Energy Secur.* 2016;5(4):212-222. doi:10.1002/fes3.96.

5. van Wijk R, van Wijk EPA. Multi-site recording and spectral analysis of spontaneous photon emission from human body. *Forsch Komplementmed.* 2005;12(2):96-106. doi:10.1159/000083766.

6. Nassarawa SS, Abdullah Sani N, Zawawi N, Ding P. Effect of light-emitting diodes (LEDs) on the quality of fruits and vegetables during postharvest period: A review. Food Bioprocess Technol. 2021;14(1):1-27.

7. Hamblin MR. Mechanisms and applications of the anti-inflammatory effects of photobiomodulation. *AIMS Biophys.* 2017;4(3):337-361. doi:10.3934/biophy.2017.3.337.

8. Pollack GH. *The Fourth Phase of Water: Beyond Solid, Liquid, and Vapor.* Seattle, WA: Ebner & Sons Publishers; 2013.

9. Brownlee M. Biochemistry and molecular cell biology of diabetic complications. *Nature.* 2001;414(6865):813-820. doi:10.1038/414813a.

10. LeGates TA, Fernandez DC, Hattar S. Light as a central modulator of circadian rhythms, sleep and affect. *Nat Rev Neurosci.* 2014;15(7):443-454. doi:10.1038/nrn3743.

11. Jain S, Hammerschlag R, Mills PJ, et al. Biofield science and healing: An emerging frontier in medicine. *Glob Adv Health Med.* 2015;4(suppl):5-7. doi:10.7453/gahmj.2015.106.suppl.

12. Wallace DC. Mitochondria and the biology of disease. *Cold Spring Harb Perspect Biol.* 2010;2(5):a004820. doi:10.1101/cshperspect.a004820.

13. McCraty R, Atkinson M, Tomasino D, Bradley RT. The coherent heart: Heart-brain interactions, psychophysiological

coherence, and the emergence of system-wide order. *Front Public Health.* 2017;5:267.

14. Kouassi KC, Koffi DM, Yao K, et al. Food quality and human health: Beyond nutrients. *Foods.* 2022;11(19):3046. doi:10.3390/foods11193046.

15. Mittelstadt BD. Principles alone cannot guarantee ethical AI. *Nat Med.* 2019;25(1):44-48. doi:10.1038/s41591-018-0315-0.

16. Maffei ME. Magnetic field effects on plant growth, development, and evolution. *Front Plant Sci.* 2014;5:445. doi:10.3389/fpls.2014.00445.

17. Reganold JP, Wachter JM. Organic agriculture in the twenty-first century. *Nat Plants.* 2016;2:15221. doi:10.1038/nplants.2015.221.

18. Prasad A, Sharma L, Yadav S, et al. Impact of postharvest handling on produce quality and nutrition. *Horticulturae.* 2020;6(4):98. doi:10.3390/horticulturae6040098.

19. Ornish D, Magbanua MJM, Weidner G, et al. Intensive lifestyle changes may affect the progression of prostate cancer. *J Urol.* 2005;174(3):1065-1069.

CHAPTER 26

Living as a Quantum Being

Embodying Light, Coherence, and Conscious Choice in Everyday Life

---

To live as a quantum being is not to reject the physical—it is to recognize that the physical is light made visible.

—James Z. Liu, MD, PhD

You Are More Than a Machine

Contemporary biology is moving away from the Newtonian view of the body as a mere biochemical machine. Evidence from biophoton research shows that every living cell emits ultra-weak photons, which serve as a communication network and coherence regulator [1,2].

To live as a quantum being means to honor this truth:

- You are not just flesh and molecules.
- You are a resonating field of light and frequency.
- Your health and longevity depend not only on nutrients and oxygen, but on the *quality of your coherence.*

Quantum living is the practice of feeding both the body and the field.

1. Cultivate Field Awareness

Begin each day not with your to-do list, but with a field check-in:

- How coherent do I feel?

- Where is energy flowing, and where is it leaking?
- What input—light, water, breath, or silence—would restore balance?

Breath and light are your first medicines, aligning autonomic rhythms and mitochondrial function [3,4].

2. Prioritize Coherence Over Productivity

In quantum biology, coherence equals efficiency [5]. Ten minutes of meditation may yield more energy and focus than hours of distracted work. A small, coherent meal may support vitality better than a large, chaotic one.

Choose actions that sustain field harmony rather than sheer output.

3. Redefine Nourishment

Nourishment is multidimensional:

- Barefoot walking under morning sunlight (circadian alignment [6]).
- Drinking structured water that holds charge and information [7].
- Breathing rhythmically to regulate HRV and vagal tone [8].
- Speaking with clarity and intention (shown to affect water and emotional states [9]).

Ask yourself: "Does this nourish my light?"

4. Listen to the Body's Light Language

Your body communicates through sensation, your field through feeling:

- Tension → incoherence.
- Ease → entrainment.

- Cravings → often signal energetic deficiency, not just nutrients.
- Fatigue → blocked light flow, not only a lack of fuel [10].

Learning to read subtle signals builds biofield literacy.

5. Design Environments That Heal

Your home, workspace, and relationships are energetic fields. Shape them to restore coherence:

- Use full-spectrum or red light after sunset to support the production of melatonin [11].
- Ground yourself in natural environments to restore electron balance [12].
- Incorporate living plants, structured water sources, and intentional soundscapes.
- Minimize EMF overload and clutter that fragments field integrity.
- Sounds of 432 Hz and 528 Hz have been shown to induce relaxation and coherence states [13].

6. Practice Radiant Responsibility

Your frequency radiates outward. Emotional coherence can positively influence others' physiological rhythms, particularly through heart–brain entrainment [14].

To embody radiant responsibility means:

- Healing for your lineage.
- Eating with awareness, knowing your choices ripple through your family field.
- Speaking with clarity, recognizing your voice as a tuning fork for coherence.

7. Align with Rhythms Greater Than You

Quantum living means recognizing your body as an extension of planetary cycles:

- Solar rhythm → circadian biology [6].
- Lunar rhythm → water cycles and emotion.
- Seasonal rhythm → nutritional patterns [15].
- Cosmic rhythm → intuition and deeper purpose.

Rhythm = coherence. Alignment with natural cycles restores vitality without force.

8. Let Stillness Become a Daily Nutrient

Silence, rest, and empty space are nutrients for the nervous system. Stillness supports signal clarity, reduces inflammation, and enhances regenerative states of the brain [16].

From stillness arises coherence. From coherence arises healing.

9. Lead by Embodied Example

You don't need to persuade others with arguments. Just live in the light.

- Let your glow be your message.
- Let your steadiness amidst chaos be your leadership.

Research on emotional contagion and social coherence shows that one person's state can influence an entire group [14]. Embodied coherence becomes silent leadership.

10. Remember Daily: You Are Light

Affirmation practice entrains identity to the field:

- "I am not only my body. I am in my field."

- "I am not just matter; I am radiant order."
- "I nourish myself with coherence, intention, and light."

Repeated intention reshapes neuroplasticity, epigenetics, and field resonance [17,18].

Final Words

To live as a quantum being is not to escape physicality; it is to inhabit fully as light made visible.

- Eat, walk, breathe, and relate as if you are already whole.
- Choose coherence over chaos.
- Align with rhythms greater than yourself.
- Lead by resonance, not persuasion.

You are coherent.
You are regeneration.
You are light.

By remembering this daily, you not only heal yourself, but you also help illuminate the path for humanity.

References

1. Popp FA, Gu Q, Li KH. Biophoton emission: Experimental background and theoretical approaches. *Mod Phys Lett B.* 1994;8(21-22):1269-1296. doi:10.1142/S0217984994001266.

2. van Wijk R, van Wijk EPA. Multi-site recording and spectral analysis of spontaneous photon emission from human body. *Forsch Komplementmed.* 2005;12(2):96-106. doi:10.1159/000083766.

3. Brown RP, Gerbarg PL. Sudarshan Kriya yogic breathing in the treatment of stress, anxiety, and depression: Part I—

Neurophysiologic model. *J Altern Complement Med.* 2005;11(1):189-201.

4. Hamblin MR. Mechanisms and applications of the anti-inflammatory effects of photobiomodulation. *AIMS Biophys.* 2017;4(3):337-361. doi:10.3934/biophy.2017.3.337.

5. Fröhlich H. Long-range coherence and energy storage in biological systems. *Int J Quantum Chem.* 1968;2(5):641-649. doi:10.1002/qua.560020505.

6. LeGates TA, Fernandez DC, Hattar S. Light as a central modulator of circadian rhythms, sleep and affect. *Nat Rev Neurosci.* 2014;15(7):443-454. doi:10.1038/nrn3743.

7. Pollack GH. *The Fourth Phase of Water: Beyond Solid, Liquid, and Vapor.* Seattle, WA: Ebner & Sons Publishers; 2013.

8. Shaffer F, McCraty R, Zerr CL. A healthy heart is not a metronome: An integrative review of the heart's anatomy and heart rate variability. *Front Psychol.* 2014;5:1040. doi:10.3389/fpsyg.2014.01040.

9. Emoto M. *The Hidden Messages in Water.* Hillsboro, OR: Beyond Words Publishing; 2005.

10. Wallace DC. Mitochondria and the biology of disease. *Cold Spring Harb Perspect Biol.* 2010;2(5):a004820. doi:10.1101/cshperspect.a004820.

11. Chang AM, Aeschbach D, Duffy JF, Czeisler CA. Evening use of light-emitting eReaders negatively affects sleep, circadian timing, and next-morning alertness. *Proc Natl Acad Sci U S A.* 2015;112(4):1232-1237. doi:10.1073/pnas.1418490112.

12. Chevalier G, Sinatra ST, Oschman JL, Delany RM. Earthing (grounding) the human body reduces blood viscosity—a major factor in cardiovascular disease. *J Altern Complement Med.* 2013;19(2):102-110. doi:10.1089/acm.2011.0820.

13. Calamassi D, Pomponi GP. Music tuned to 440 Hz versus 432 Hz and the health effects: A double-blind cross-over pilot study. *Explore (NY).* 2019;15(4):283-290. doi:10.1016/j.explore.2019.01.001.

14. McCraty R, Atkinson M, Tomasino D, Bradley RT. The coherent heart: Heart-brain interactions, psychophysiological coherence, and the emergence of system-wide order. *Front Public Health.* 2017;5:267.

15. Mattson MP, Allison DB, Fontana L, et al. Meal frequency and timing in health and disease. *Proc Natl Acad Sci U S A.* 2014;111(47):16647-16653. doi:10.1073/pnas.1413965111.

16. Tang YY, Hölzel BK, Posner MI. The neuroscience of mindfulness meditation. *Nat Rev Neurosci.* 2015;16(4):213-225. doi:10.1038/nrn3916.

17. Ornish D, Lin J, Daubenmier J, et al. Increased telomerase activity and comprehensive lifestyle changes: A pilot study. *Lancet Oncol.* 2008;9(11):1048-1057. doi:10.1016/S1470-2045(08)70234-1.

18. Davidson RJ, Kabat-Zinn J, Schumacher J, et al. Alterations in brain and immune function produced by mindfulness meditation. *Psychosom Med.* 2003;65(4):564-570. doi:10.1097/01.PSY.0000077505.67574.E3.

CHAPTER 27

Mitochondrial Deficiency Is a Kind of Biophoton Deficiency

Why Many Diseases Caused by Mitochondrial Dysfunction Can Be Treated with a Biophoton Generator

---

When mitochondria are starving, it's not just fuel they lack—it's light. **—James Z. Liu, MD, PhD**

Mitochondria as Quantum Antennas

Mitochondria are often described as the "powerhouses of the cell" because of their role in ATP production through oxidative phosphorylation. But this reductionist metaphor misses their quantum biological role: mitochondria are light-sensitive bio-antennae that regulate not only energy but also coherence, communication, and regeneration.

Key insights from biophoton research show:

- Living cells emit ultraweak photon emissions (biophotons) during metabolic activity [1].
- Mitochondria are a primary source of these emissions, especially during oxidative phosphorylation [2].
- Biophoton emission correlates with cellular order, DNA repair, and mitochondrial vitality [3].
- Mitochondria also respond to external light, particularly in the red and near-infrared spectrum (600–950 nm), which enhances their function [4].

Thus, mitochondria are not just engines; they are gateways between biochemical metabolism and the quantum field of light.

When Mitochondria Lose Light

Mitochondrial dysfunction is a hallmark of many chronic diseases. Traditionally, this has been described in terms of:

- Decreased ATP production
- Oxidative stress and ROS overload
- Impaired detoxification and apoptosis

But from a quantum perspective, the core issue is biophoton deficiency: mitochondria lose their ability to emit coherent light, leading to loss of cellular communication, field order, and systemic vitality [1,5].

Conditions linked to mitochondrial and biophoton deficiency include:

- Neurodegenerative diseases (Alzheimer's, Parkinson's) [6–10]
- Metabolic syndrome and type 2 diabetes [11–14]
- Chronic fatigue syndrome (ME/CFS) and fibromyalgia [15]
- Autoimmune disorders [16]
- Cardiovascular disease [17]
- Certain cancers, where mitochondrial signaling is disrupted [18–20]

In each case, disease is not only an energy crisis but also a loss of intracellular light.

Biophoton Generators as Mitochondrial Support

Biophoton generators emit coherent, biologically active light fields that can entrain cells back into order. Unlike isolated laser therapies, generators create a sustained ambient photonic environment, often applied passively during sleep.

Effects on mitochondrial recovery include:

- Re-energizing respiration by enhancing cytochrome c oxidase activity (critical for ATP synthesis) [4,21].
- Reducing oxidative stress by improving electron flow efficiency.
- Enhancing intracellular communication by restoring photon coherence.
- Promoting stem cell activation and tissue regeneration [22,23].

Clinical Observations

Alzheimer's and Dementia

Red/NIR light has been shown to improve cognition in neurodegenerative models [6]. Case reports with overnight biophoton exposure show:

- Sharper recall
- Reduced agitation
- Improved sleep quality

Chronic Pain and Inflammation

Photobiomodulation reduces nerve inflammation and musculoskeletal pain [12]. Biophoton therapy enhances:

- Mobility
- Pain relief without drugs
- Faster wound healing

Type 2 Diabetes

Structured light exposure supports:

- Better glucose metabolism [7,12–14]
- Reduced neuropathic pain
- Improved pancreatic mitochondrial activity

Stroke Recovery

Red/NIR light accelerates neuroplasticity after traumatic brain injury [24]. Biophoton generators extend this by:

- Supporting mitochondrial repair in ischemic tissue
- Enhancing motor recovery [25,26].

Why Biophoton Therapy Works Where Drugs Struggle

Pharmaceuticals typically:

- Suppress symptoms
- Block pathways
- Add metabolic burden

By contrast, biophoton therapy:

- Restores the signal (light coherence)
- Restructures the field (bioelectromagnetic order)
- Activates self-healing (autophagy, stem cells)
- Works holistically, not selectively

The result is true reversal rather than symptom management.

Mitochondria as Photonic Gateways

Mitochondria are more than ATP producers. They are transducers of universal light—interfaces between the quantum field and biological form.

- When they shine, we thrive.
- When they dim, disease takes hold.
- When fed coherent photons, they remember how to regenerate.

Summary: A New Paradigm of Healing

Old View	Quantum View
Mitochondria make ATP	Mitochondria regulate light, order, and communication
Disease = chemical dysfunction	Disease = loss of coherence and photon deficiency
Treatment = suppression	Treatment = restoring light-based order

To heal is to restore the intracellular light that organizes life.
To reverse chronic disease is to treat biophoton deficiency at its core.
To live vibrantly is to remember: *you are a being of light—feed the light, especially within your cells.*

Reference

1. Popp FA. Biophotons—background, experimental results, theoretical approach and applications. In: Popp FA, Beloussov LV, eds. *Integrative Biophysics: Biophotonics.* Dordrecht, Netherlands: Springer; 2003:387-438. doi:10.1007/978-94-017-0373-4_12.

2. Kobayashi M, Takeda M, Sato T, et al. In vivo imaging of spontaneous ultraweak photon emission from a rat's brain correlated with cerebral energy metabolism and oxidative stress. *Neuroreport.* 1999;10(4):875-879.

3. van Wijk R, van Wijk EPA. Multi-site recording and spectral analysis of spontaneous photon emission from human body. *Forsch Komplementmed.* 2005;12(2):96-106.

4. Hamblin MR. Mechanisms and applications of the anti-inflammatory effects of photobiomodulation. *AIMS Biophys.* 2017;4(3):337-361. doi:10.3934/biophy.2017.3.337.

5. Zapata F, Fernández-Ruiz R, González D, et al. Human ultra-weak photon emission as non-invasive spectroscopic tool for diagnosis of internal states: A review. *J Photochem Photobiol B.* 2021;216:112141.

6. Hamblin MR. Photobiomodulation for Alzheimer's disease and other dementias. *J Alzheimers Dis.* 2016;55(3):923-933. doi:10.3233/JAD-160348.

7. Liu JZ, Smotrys M, Robinson SD, Liu S, Gu HY. Therapeutic benefits of biophoton therapy in Parkinson's disease: Clinical evidence from a pilot and real-world study. *J Neurol Res Rev Rep.* 2025;7(6):1-6.

8. Liu JZ, Smotrys MA, Robinson SD, Yu HX, Liu SX, Liu DR, Gu HY. Quantitative EEG evidence of functional brain recovery in Parkinson's disease following biophoton therapy. *J Neurol Res Rev Rep.* 2025;7(7):14-20.

9. Liu JZ, Smotrys MA, Robinson SD, Yu HX, Liu SX, Liu DR, Gu HY. Multimodal evidence of cognitive restoration in Alzheimer's disease following biophoton therapy: A neurophysiological and energetic assessment. *J Alzheimers Dis Rep.* 2025;2(3):1-10. doi:10.47363/JADR/2025(2)107.

10. Liu JZ, Smotrys MA, Robinson SD, Yu HX, Liu SX, Liu DR, Gu HY. Quantitative EEG evidence of cognitive restoration

in Alzheimer's disease following biophoton generator therapy. *J Neurol Res Rev Rep.* 2025;7(7):1-7.

11. Type 2 Diabetes Petersen KF, Dufour S, Befroy D, Garcia R, Shulman GI. Impaired mitochondrial activity in the insulin-resistant offspring of patients with type 2 diabetes. *N Engl J Med.* 2004;350(7):664-671.

12. Hu Y, Gu HY, Liu JZ. Reversal of tissue glycation and cholesterol accumulation by strong biophotons: A new anti-aging mechanism. *Gerontol Geriatr Stud.* 2025;9(3):715.

13. Hu Y, Gu HY, Liu JZ. Progressive blood morphology restoration in a diabetic patient using biophoton therapy: A live blood-cell analysis over six weeks. *J Diabetes Res Rev Rep.* 2025, 7(4): 1-5.

14. Myhill S, Booth NE, McLaren-Howard J. Chronic fatigue syndrome and mitochondrial dysfunction. *Int J Clin Exp Med.* 2009;2(1):1-16.

15. Staal J, Beyaert R, et al. Editorial: Mitochondrial dysfunction in inflammation and autoimmunity. *Front Immunol.* 2023;14:1304315. doi:10.3389/fimmu.2023.1304315.

16. Madamanchi NR, Vendrov A, Runge MS. Oxidative stress and vascular disease. *Arterioscler Thromb Vasc Biol.* 2005;25(1):29-38. doi:10.1161/01.ATV.0000150649.39934.13.

17. Wallace DC. Mitochondria and cancer. *Nat Rev Cancer.* 2012;12(10):685-698. doi:10.1038/nrc3365.

18. Liu JZ, Ramirez AD, Osborn K, Osborn L, Ager A, Gu HY. Biophoton quantum therapy enabled cancer treatments to reach their utmost goal of cancer-free. *Gerontol Geriatr Stud.* 2025;9(4):718. doi:10.31031/GGS.2025.09.000718.

19. Hu Y, Gu HY, Liu JZ. Strong biophoton field therapy as a quantum adjunct to enhance cancer recovery: A live blood microscopy case study with clinical correlation. *Biomed J Sci Tech Res.* 2025;62(2):9724.

20. Chung H, Dai T, Sharma SK, Huang YY, Carroll JD, Hamblin MR. The nuts and bolts of low-level laser (light) therapy. *Ann Biomed Eng.* 2012;40(2):516-533. doi:10.1007/s10439-011-0454-7.

21. Basso FG, Oliveira CF, Kurachi C, et al. Low-level laser therapy for osteogenic differentiation of dental pulp stem cells. *J Endod.* 2016;42(2):275-280. doi:10.1016/j.joen.2015.10.012.

22. Liu JZ, Smotrys MA, Robinson SD, Yu HX, Liu SX, Liu DR, Gu HY. Biophoton-driven stem cell activation: Revolutionary non-invasive approach to regenerative medicine and anti-aging. Keynote presentation presented at: The 2nd World Conference on Aging and Gerontology; July 14-15, 2025; Rome, Italy.

23. Liu JZ, Gu HY. Biophoton quantum physical medicine to treat severe chronic pain – a non-drug therapy. Keynote presentation presented at: *Advances in Addiction Medicine and Mental Health*; June 24, 2025; Berlin, Germany.

24. Xuan W, Vatansever F, Huang L, et al. Transcranial low-level laser therapy improves neurological performance in traumatic brain injury in mice: Effect of treatment repetition regimen. *J Biomed Opt.* 2013;18(9):098003.

25. Liu JZ, Smotrys MA, Robinson SD, Yu HX, Liu SX, Liu DR, Gu HY. Biophoton therapy reverses electrophysiological

deficits in chronic traumatic brain injury: Quantitative EEG evidence of cognitive and network recovery. *J Neurol Res Rev Rep*. 2025;7(8):1-11.

26. Thomas T, Gu HY, Smotrys MA, Robinson SD, Liu JZ. Non-invasive biophoton therapy for neurocognitive and physical recovery in retired athletes with traumatic brain injury: A pilot study in former NFL players. J Neurol Res Rev Rep, 2025, 7(8): 2-6.

CHAPTER 28

Biophoton Deficiency and Lack of Coherence Are the Causes of the Most Common Disorders

From Quantum Signaling Failure to Systemic Physiological Imbalance

---

Disease is not merely a chemical imbalance—it is a loss of light, a breakdown in coherence.

—James Z. Liu, MD, PhD

Introduction

Modern medicine explains disease largely in terms of biochemistry and genetics, yet increasing evidence from biophotonics and quantum biology suggests that disorders also emerge from a more fundamental level: a loss of cellular light emission and field coherence.

Healthy cells generate ultra-weak photon emissions (biophotons) during metabolic activity, particularly within the mitochondria. These biophotons are not random "by-products" but act as regulatory signals coordinating DNA activity, enzymatic reactions, and cell-to-cell communication [1,2].

When biophoton production declines through aging, stress, toxicity, or chronic inflammation, the body loses the coherence necessary for systemic regulation. This deficiency manifests clinically as the most common disorders of modern life: neurodegenerative disease, metabolic dysfunction, cardiovascular disorders, immune dysregulation, and chronic fatigue.

Biophoton Deficiency as a Core Mechanism

1. Mitochondrial Dysfunction and Energy Loss

Mitochondria are the main source of both ATP and biophotons. During oxidative phosphorylation, coherent photon emissions synchronize metabolic pathways [3]. In disease states such as Parkinson's, Alzheimer's, or diabetes, mitochondrial activity declines, ATP falls, and photon output diminishes. This leads to cellular "noise" and poor regulation.

- Evidence: Reduced photon emission has been observed in stressed, inflamed, and cancerous cells compared to healthy controls [4].
- Clinical consequences: Fatigue, neurodegeneration, and immune system weakness are associated with this light deficiency.

2. Loss of Coherence in Cellular Communication

Biophotons act as a communication network, enabling coordination beyond chemical diffusion. The German biophysicist Fritz-Albert Popp demonstrated that healthy systems emit coherent light, whereas diseased systems show chaotic, noisy emissions [1].

- In cancer, cells emit chaotic, uncoordinated photons, reflecting loss of regulatory order.
- In cardiovascular disease, disrupted electromagnetic fields reduce vascular and autonomic coherence, contributing to arrhythmias and hypertension [5].

3. Oxidative Stress and Inflammation

Excessive reactive oxygen species (ROS) disrupt mitochondrial metabolism and alter photon emissions. Chronic oxidative stress leads to "dimmer" cells with distorted resonance patterns [6].

- Disorders linked: Diabetes, atherosclerosis, arthritis, and neurodegeneration.
- Biophoton deficiency here reflects signal breakdown in addition to structural damage.

4. Environmental and Lifestyle Disruptions

- Artificial EMFs interfere with natural biophoton signaling [7].
- Poor diet (processed foods lacking coherent light) reduces photonic intake.
- Sleep deprivation disrupts melatonin rhythms and photon-mediated DNA repair [8].

Together, these contribute to a chronic mismatch between internal biofields and external natural rhythms.

Common Disorders Rooted in Biophoton Deficiency

1. Neurodegenerative Diseases

Alzheimer's and Parkinson's disease are characterized by mitochondrial decline, oxidative stress, and disrupted neural coherence. Photobiomodulation studies show that red/NIR light can restore mitochondrial ATP and biophoton activity, thereby improving cognition [9].

2. Metabolic Syndrome and Diabetes

Insulin resistance involves mitochondrial inefficiency and ROS burden, both of which lower photon emission. Biophoton support improves cellular energy flow, aiding glucose regulation [10].

3. Cardiovascular Disorders

Heart rate variability (HRV), a measure of systemic coherence, is reduced in heart disease. Biophoton deficiency contributes to poor vascular communication and energy depletion [11]. Hence, biophoton deficiency directly links to the occurrence of heart disease.

4. Immune Dysfunction

Low coherence disrupts immune cell signaling, contributing to the development of autoimmune or chronic infections. Studies suggest that photobiomodulation improves immune regulation through enhanced mitochondrial function [12].

5. Chronic Fatigue and Depression

These conditions reflect global energy deficiency at both the mitochondrial and field levels. Light therapy increases coherence, improving mood, focus, and endurance [13].

Mechanistic Summary

Pathway	Biophoton Role	Effect of Deficiency	Clinical Outcome
Mitochondria	Generate ATP + photons	Energy + light loss	Fatigue, neurodegeneration
DNA signaling	Photon-guided transcription	Miscommunication	Cancer, autoimmunity
Immune system	Light coordinates response	Chaotic defense	Chronic infection, inflammation
Nervous system	Coherent oscillations	Disrupted coherence	Depression, Alzheimer's

Toward Coherence-Based Medicine

Biophoton therapy, via red/NIR light, structured water, coherent foods, and biophoton generators, offers a path to restore light and order where drugs alone cannot.

- It enhances mitochondrial ATP and photon emission.
- Rebuilds coherence across organs and systems.
- Supports self-regulation and repair rather than symptom suppression.

By reframing the most common disorders as manifestations of biophoton deficiency, medicine can move toward a model of restoration instead of suppression.

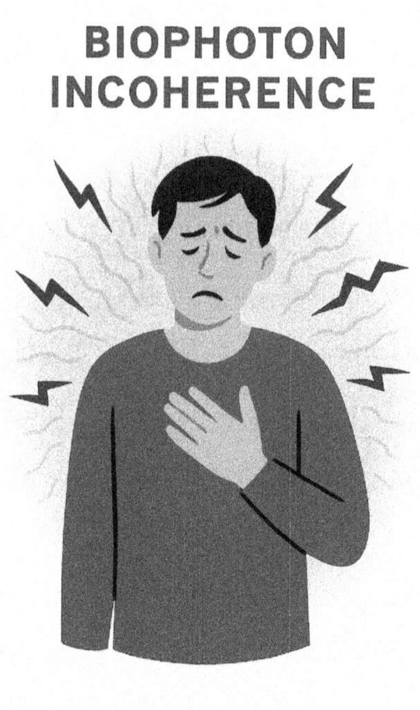

Figure 28.1. Biophoton Incoherence and Sickness. *Illustration of biophoton incoherence, where disrupted and chaotic energy patterns around the body are associated with imbalance, stress, and sickness. The disordered field reflects a loss of harmony in cellular communication and reduced vitality.*

Conclusion

The most prevalent modern disorders—neurodegeneration, metabolic disease, cardiovascular dysfunction, immune dysregulation, and chronic fatigue—can all be understood as consequences of lost biophoton emission and systemic incoherence.

Health is light. Disease is dimming.
By feeding and restoring our light, coherence returns, and with it, the possibility of true healing.

References

1. Popp FA. About the coherence of biophotons. *Macroscopic Quantum Coherence.* 1998;1(1):1–6.
2. van Wijk R. Biophotons and biocommunication. *J Sci Explor.* 2014;28(1):43–62.
3. Karu TI. Mitochondrial signaling activated by red and near-IR radiation. *Photochem Photobiol.* 2008;84(5):1091–1099.
4. Tang R, Dai J. Biophoton signal transmission and biological function. *Sci China Life Sci.* 2014;57(7):726–740.
5. McCraty R, Shaffer F. Heart rate variability: new perspectives on physiological mechanisms, assessment, and biofeedback. *Front Psychol.* 2015;6:55.
6. Mittler R. Oxidative stress, antioxidants, and stress tolerance in plants and humans. *Trends Plant Sci.* 2002;7(9):405–410.
7. Pall ML. Electromagnetic fields act via activation of voltage-gated calcium channels. *J Cell Mol Med.* 2013;17(8):958–965.
8. Kennaway DJ and Wright H. Melatonin and circadian rhythms. *Curr Top Med Chem.* 2002 Feb;2(2):199–209.

9. Salehpour F, Cassano P. Transcranial photobiomodulation therapy for cognitive impairment: a systematic review. *Neurophotonics.* 2021;8(2):022001.

10. Hamblin MR. Photobiomodulation for diabetes and related complications. *World J Diabetes.* 2022;13(2):80–94.

11. Shaffer F, McCraty R. Coherence: bridging personal, social, and global health. *Glob Adv Health Med.* 2016;5(1):82–90.

12. Farivar S, Malekshahabi T, Shiari R. Biological effects of low-level laser therapy. *Lasers Med Sci.* 2014;29(2):559–566.

13. Kinjo M, et al. Transcranial magnetic stimulation neurophysiology of patients with major depressive disorder: a systematic review and meta-analysis. *Psychol Med.* 2020 Dec 3;51(1):1–10. doi: 10.1017/S0033291720004729

PART IV

Commercial Usages of Biophoton Quantum Nutrition

Part IV explores how the principles of Biophoton Quantum Nutrition extend beyond individual wellness to encompass large-scale, commercial, and societal applications. Here, light and coherence are positioned not only as tools for personal health but also as transformative assets for education, sports, agriculture, food industries, and even pharmaceuticals.

Chapter 29 highlights the role of biophotons in *enhancing student learning and academic performance,* improving memory, focus, and resilience under exam stress.

Chapter 30 demonstrates how biophoton energy can *reduce fatigue and optimize workplace productivity,* offering a drug-free solution for burnout and cognitive overload.

Chapter 31 applies quantum nutrition to *athletic performance,* showing how light-based interventions boost endurance, recovery, and mental focus for competitive advantage.

Chapter 32 extends this to equine sports, where *horse racing performance* is improved through faster recovery, stronger connective tissues, and greater stamina.

Chapter 33 addresses the food supply chain, revealing how biophoton energy *enhances the freshness, nutritional value, and safety* of produce without reliance on chemical preservatives.

Chapter 34 expands into agriculture, presenting evidence that biophotons *increase yield and nutrient density in high-value crops,* while also enhancing resilience to stress and disease.

Chapter 35 explores applications in the *wine industry*, where biophoton-enhanced fermentation accelerates yeast metabolism, improves flavor complexity, and stabilizes product quality.

Chapter 36 examines the *pharmaceutical sector*, showing how biophoton energy improves microbial and cell-culture fermentation, boosting yields of antibiotics, vaccines, biologics, and enzymes.

Together, these chapters reveal the vast commercial potential of Biophoton Quantum Nutrition. From classrooms to sports arenas, farms to laboratories, and vineyards to bioreactors, light emerges as a universal enhancer of performance, productivity, and quality. This section demonstrates that the same principles that heal individuals can also revolutionize industries, reshaping global health, food security, and economic sustainability.

The Broader Vision

Part V illustrates that biophotons are not confined to clinical or personal wellness—they are foundational to industrial ecology and agriculture. By embedding quantum nutrition principles into food systems and production cycles, humanity can move toward:

- Eco-conscious industries minimize waste and energy.
- Healthier foods that carry higher photonic vitality to consumers.
- Resilient supply chains that are less vulnerable to spoilage, resource scarcity, and climate disruptions.

In summary, Part IV demonstrates that Biophoton Quantum Nutrition is not only a personal practice but also a commercially and societally innovative, scalable, sustainable, and transformative approach to agriculture and industry that aligns human vitality with planetary well-being.

CHAPTER 29

Biophotons Increase Students' Learning and Testing Performances

From Brain Fog to Brilliance: The Photonic Path to Academic Excellence

---

By enhancing mitochondrial energy and neural coherence, biophotons offer a new pathway to optimize focus, memory, and mental endurance—empowering students to learn more efficiently and perform at their highest potential.

—James Z. Liu, MD, PhD

Introduction

Academic achievement depends not only on knowledge but also on cognitive efficiency, sustained attention, stress resilience, and psychological balance. In the modern educational environment, students face unprecedented information overload, prolonged study hours, and heightened exam pressures, all of which contribute to mental fatigue, impaired learning, and reduced test performance.

Conventional approaches such as nootropic drugs, dietary supplements, and cognitive training provide partial benefits but often carry risks, side effects, or inconsistent results. Biophoton therapy—non-invasive modulation of cellular and neural activity using ultraweak or low-level light—offers a promising complementary method for optimizing cognition, memory, and stress resilience in students.

Challenges in Modern Education

- Cognitive overload: Rapid exposure to vast information diminishes comprehension and long-term retention.
- Mental fatigue: Prolonged study reduces neuronal energy reserves, impairing learning efficiency.
- Stress and anxiety: Elevated cortisol disrupts hippocampal activity, undermining memory and executive function.
- Attention deficits: Reduced neural coherence shortens focus spans, limiting productivity.

Biophoton Mechanisms in Optimizing Learning

1. Enhancement of Cognitive Function

- Biophoton exposure stimulates neuronal excitability and synaptic plasticity, accelerating processing speed and mental clarity [1,2].
- Long-term potentiation (LTP), a key mechanism of learning and memory, improves under light stimulation [2].

2. Reduction of Mental Fatigue

- By stimulating mitochondrial cytochrome c oxidase, red and near-infrared (NIR) light enhances ATP synthesis, sustaining neuronal energy [1,3].
- Students report increased study endurance during intensive sessions with light-based support.

3. Improved Focus and Attention

- Light therapy modulates neurotransmitters such as dopamine and serotonin, essential for focus and emotional regulation [4].

- Enhanced brainwave coherence reduces distractibility and strengthens deep-focus states.

4. Stress Regulation

- Biophoton stimulation influences the autonomic nervous system, lowering cortisol while enhancing parasympathetic tone [5].
- This promotes calmness, resilience, and improved performance under exam pressure.

5. Memory Retention and Recall

- Light therapy improves cerebral blood flow and oxygen delivery to the hippocampus, enhancing memory encoding and retrieval [6].
- Optimized neurovascular coupling supports sharper recall during testing situations.

Mechanistic Summary

- Neuroplasticity Enhancement: Facilitates the formation of new neuronal pathways for learning.
- Mitochondrial Optimization: Sustains ATP supply for prolonged cognitive tasks.
- Anti-inflammatory Effects: Reduces neuroinflammation that interferes with executive function.
- Improved Cerebral Circulation: Supports nutrient and oxygen delivery to learning centers.

Observed Outcomes in Students

Students and pilot educational studies integrating biophoton therapies report:

- Higher Test Scores: Linked to improved recall, problem-solving, and focus.

- Faster Learning Speed: Quicker assimilation of new concepts.
- Reduced Test Anxiety: Emotional calmness during exams.
- Better Mental Health: Lower stress, improved sleep, and greater emotional balance.

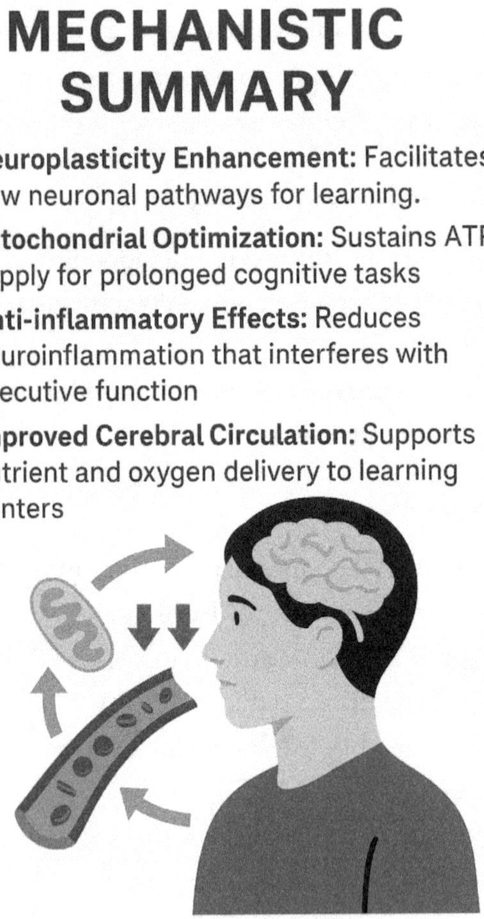

Figure 29.1. Biophotons Improve Learning Ability. *Mechanistic summary of cognitive enhancement. Neuroplasticity enhancement facilitates the formation of new neuronal pathways, mitochondrial optimization sustains ATP supply for cognitive tasks, anti-inflammatory effects reduce neuroinflammation, and improved cerebral circulation supports nutrient and oxygen delivery to learning centers.*

Integration into Educational Systems

- In-Class Use: Installing biophoton generators or light therapy devices in classrooms to enhance group learning environments.
- Personal Study Devices: Portable units for focused concentration at home.
- After-School Programs: Biophoton exposure during tutoring or exam-preparation sessions.

Policy and Research Recommendations

- Controlled Trials: Randomized studies to evaluate effects on learning, memory, and exam performance.
- Holistic Integration: Combine biophoton therapy with sleep hygiene, nutrition, and mindfulness practices.
- Awareness Campaigns: Educate parents, teachers, and policymakers on safe, evidence-informed applications.

Conclusion

Biophoton therapy represents a transformative adjunct in education. By enhancing synaptic plasticity, mitochondrial health, cerebral circulation, and autonomic balance, it supports the core capacities students need for academic excellence. Unlike pharmacological aids, it is non-invasive, safe, and field-oriented, working with the body's natural information systems.

As future educational models embrace biophoton-rich environments, schools could evolve into coherent learning ecosystems—where stress is minimized, memory is maximized, and students thrive as radiant learners.

References

1. Karu T. Mitochondrial signaling in mammalian cells activated by red and near-IR radiation. *Photochem Photobiol.* 2008;84(5):1091–1099.

2. Hamblin MR. Mechanisms of low-level light therapy. *Proc SPIE.* 2009;7165:716502.

3. Chung H, et al. The nuts and bolts of low-level laser (light) therapy. *Ann Biomed Eng.* 2012;40(2):516–533.

4. Salehpour F, Cassano P. Transcranial photobiomodulation therapy for cognitive impairment: a systematic review. *Neurophotonics.* 2021;8(2):022001.

5. Kinjo M et al. Transcranial magnetic stimulation neurophysiology of patients with major depressive disorder: a systematic review and meta-analysis. *Psychol Med.* 2020 Dec 3;51(1):1–10.

6. Henderson TA, Morries LD. Near-infrared photonic energy penetration: Can infrared phototherapy effectively reach the human brain? *Neuropsychiatr Dis Treat.* 2015;11:2191–2208.

CHAPTER 30

Biophoton Energy Reduces Fatigue and Improves Working Performance

Recharging the Human System: Light, Vitality, and Peak Output

---

Fatigue is not the absence of strength, but the loss of order in the light within.

—James Z. Liu, MD, PhD

Introduction

Fatigue is one of the most common barriers to productivity and well-being. It manifests as persistent tiredness, weakness, and lack of motivation, impairing both mental and physical performance. Traditional strategies such as rest, nutrition, and stress reduction are essential but often fail to deliver sustained relief, especially in high-demand work, academic, and clinical environments.

Biophoton therapy—low-level exposure to coherent light fields—offers a non-invasive, drug-free approach to reducing fatigue. By enhancing mitochondrial efficiency, circulation, neural coherence, and circadian regulation, biophoton stimulation has shown potential to restore energy, resilience, and cognitive performance [1–3].

Understanding Fatigue and Work Performance

Types of Fatigue

- Physical Fatigue: Caused by prolonged exertion or inadequate recovery; reduces muscular endurance.
- Mental Fatigue: Characterized by cognitive slowing, reduced memory, and poor decision-making.
- Chronic Fatigue: Persistent exhaustion linked to mitochondrial dysfunction, inflammation, or neurological imbalance.

Impact on Productivity

- Lower efficiency and increased workplace errors.
- Reduced motivation, creativity, and problem-solving.
- Greater risk of burnout, absenteeism, and accidents.

Biophoton Mechanisms in Reducing Fatigue

1. Boosting Cellular Energy Production

- Red and near-infrared (NIR) light stimulates cytochrome c oxidase, the terminal enzyme in the mitochondrial respiratory chain [1, 2].
- It enhances ATP synthesis, providing sustained energy for muscles and neurons.

2. Enhancing Oxygenation and Circulation

- Biophoton exposure improves microvascular blood flow and oxygen delivery [3].
- Enhanced perfusion supports both physical endurance and cognitive alertness.

3. Regulating Neurotransmitter Activity

- Photobiomodulation influences dopamine and serotonin pathways, critical for motivation, focus, and mood [4].
- Improved neurotransmission reduces distractibility and supports task engagement.

4. Reducing Oxidative Stress and Inflammation

- Light therapy upregulates antioxidant enzymes and reduces reactive oxygen species (ROS) [5].
- Lower oxidative stress improves resilience and recovery capacity.

5. Balancing Hormonal Function

- Biophoton exposure modulates cortisol rhythms and promotes endorphin release.
- This supports stress resilience and sustained vitality.

6. Improving Sleep Quality

- Photobiomodulation helps regulate the circadian clock and enhances melatonin secretion [6].
- Improved sleep efficiency reduces fatigue and sharpens mental clarity.

Applications in Daily Life and Work

- Corporate Wellness: On-site biophoton generators reduce burnout and absenteeism.
- Athletic Performance: Accelerates recovery, reduces lactate accumulation, and enhances endurance.
- Academic Settings: Improves focus and mental endurance during study and exams.

- Shift Work and Healthcare: Supports irregular schedules by restoring circadian balance and energy.

Scientific Insights

- Mitochondrial Efficiency: Increased ATP supports sustained muscle and brain activity [1,2].
- Cognitive Function: Faster processing speed and reaction time under light exposure [4].
- Muscle Recovery: Reduced lactate accumulation improves endurance [3].
- Circadian Alignment: Improved synchronization of biological rhythms supports alertness [6].

Case Studies and Observations

- Workplace: Employees using biophoton therapy reported reduced brain fog and improved productivity.
- Athletics: Athletes noted faster recovery and enhanced training capacity.
- Healthcare Workers: Reported greater focus, reduced stress, and better sleep despite night shifts.

Integration into Routines

- Morning Activation: Red/NIR sessions to boost mitochondrial charge and focus.
- Midday Recharge: Short sessions counteract afternoon fatigue.
- Post-Work Recovery: Evening therapy reduces stress accumulation.
- Portable Devices: Enable continuous support in offices, homes, and during travel.

Future Research and Innovations

- Performance Trials: Assessing effects on productivity, reaction time, and workplace safety.
- Occupational Health: Evaluating reductions in burnout and stress biomarkers.
- Wearable Devices: Integrating biophoton emitters into headbands or clothing for real-time support.
- Global Access: Adoption into corporate wellness and public health fatigue-management strategies.

Ethical Considerations

- Biophoton therapy is non-invasive, safe, and drug-free, with no reported adverse effects [2,5].
- It should complement—not replace—healthy lifestyle practices such as rest, movement, and nutrition.

Conclusion

Biophoton therapy represents a transformative approach to managing fatigue and optimizing performance. By recharging mitochondria, improving circulation, modulating neurotransmitters, and supporting circadian balance, it offers sustained energy without the risks associated with stimulants or pharmaceuticals.

From offices to athletic fields, classrooms to clinics, biophoton technologies can reshape how society addresses fatigue, empowering individuals to work, learn, and live with greater vitality.

References

1. Karu T. Mitochondrial signaling in mammalian cells activated by red and near-IR radiation. *Photochem Photobiol.* 2008;84(5):1091–1099.

2. Hamblin MR. Mechanisms of photobiomodulation in human cells. *J Biophotonics.* 2017;10(11):1462–1481.

3. Wong-Riley MT, et al. Photobiomodulation directly benefits primary neurons functionally inactivated by toxins. *J Biol Chem.* 2005;280(6):4761–4771.

4. Salehpour F, Cassano P. Transcranial photobiomodulation therapy for cognitive enhancement. *Neurophotonics.* 2021;8(2):022001.

5. Gao X, Xing D. Molecular mechanisms of cell proliferation induced by photobiomodulation. *J Biomed Sci.* 2009;16:4.

6. Gaggi NL, Parincu Z, Peterson A, O'Brien C, Kam K, Tural U, et al. Enhancing sleep, wakefulness, and cognition with transcranial photobiomodulation: a systematic review. *Front. Behav. Neurosci.* 2025;19:1542462. doi:10.3389/fnbeh.2025.1542462.

CHAPTER 31

Biophotons Energize Athletes to Improve Competitiveness

Optimizing Biological Coherence for Strength, Endurance, and Competitive Edge

---

When internal light is ordered, the body expresses power effortlessly.
—James Z. Liu, MD, PhD

Introduction

Athletic performance is determined not only by physical conditioning but also by psychological resilience, recovery efficiency, and cellular energy capacity. Despite advances in sports nutrition, strength training, and recovery science, many athletes still struggle with fatigue, delayed recovery, and inconsistent performance.

Biophoton therapy, based on the application of red and near-infrared (NIR) light to stimulate cellular bioenergetics, represents a safe, non-invasive, and performance-enhancing technology. By optimizing mitochondrial activity, accelerating tissue repair, reducing inflammation, and supporting mental clarity, biophoton therapy provides athletes with a novel method to gain a competitive edge [1,2].

The Demands of Competitive Sports

- Physical Strain: Intense training induces microtrauma, oxidative stress, and metabolic fatigue that limit performance.
- Mental Pressure: Competitive events require sustained concentration, emotional control, and resilience to stress.
- Recovery Needs: Rapid restoration between training sessions and competitions is essential for maintaining consistency.
- Injury Risk: Heavy workloads increase the likelihood of musculoskeletal injuries and overtraining syndrome.

Why Biophoton Therapy Benefits Athletes

1. Enhances Cellular Energy Production

- Red/NIR light stimulates cytochrome c oxidase in the mitochondrial respiratory chain [1,2].
- This increases ATP output, improving endurance, power, and sustained intensity.

2. Accelerates Recovery

- Biophoton therapy modulates inflammatory cytokines (IL-6, TNF-α), reducing tissue damage and pain [3].
- Stimulates fibroblast activity and collagen synthesis, facilitating muscle and joint repair after strenuous sessions.

3. Improves Oxygen Utilization

- Enhances microcirculation and hemorheology, delivering oxygen and nutrients to active muscles more efficiently [4].
- Supports aerobic metabolism, delays the onset of fatigue, and improves VO_2 max capacity.

4. Reduces Muscle Fatigue and Soreness

- Improves lactate clearance and reduces oxidative stress, thereby minimizing delayed-onset muscle soreness (DOMS) [5].
- Enables higher training frequency without loss of performance quality.

5. Strengthens Mental Focus and Stress Resilience

- Modulates dopamine and serotonin pathways, enhancing mental clarity and emotional stability [6].
- Supports quicker reaction times, concentration, and decision-making under pressure.

6. Supports Injury Prevention and Rehabilitation

- Promotes musculoskeletal resilience by strengthening connective tissues.
- Enhances recovery from sprains, strains, or fractures, reducing downtime and recurrence.

Mechanisms of Action for Athletic Performance

- Mitochondrial Optimization: Improves cellular energy metabolism and delays fatigue.
- Anti-Inflammatory Modulation: Reduces the risk of overtraining and accelerates tissue recovery.
- Improved Circulation: Enhances oxygen delivery and nutrient transport to muscles.
- Neuroregulation: Sharpens focus, coordination, and reflexes.
- Hormonal Balance: Supports growth factor activity and stress hormone regulation.

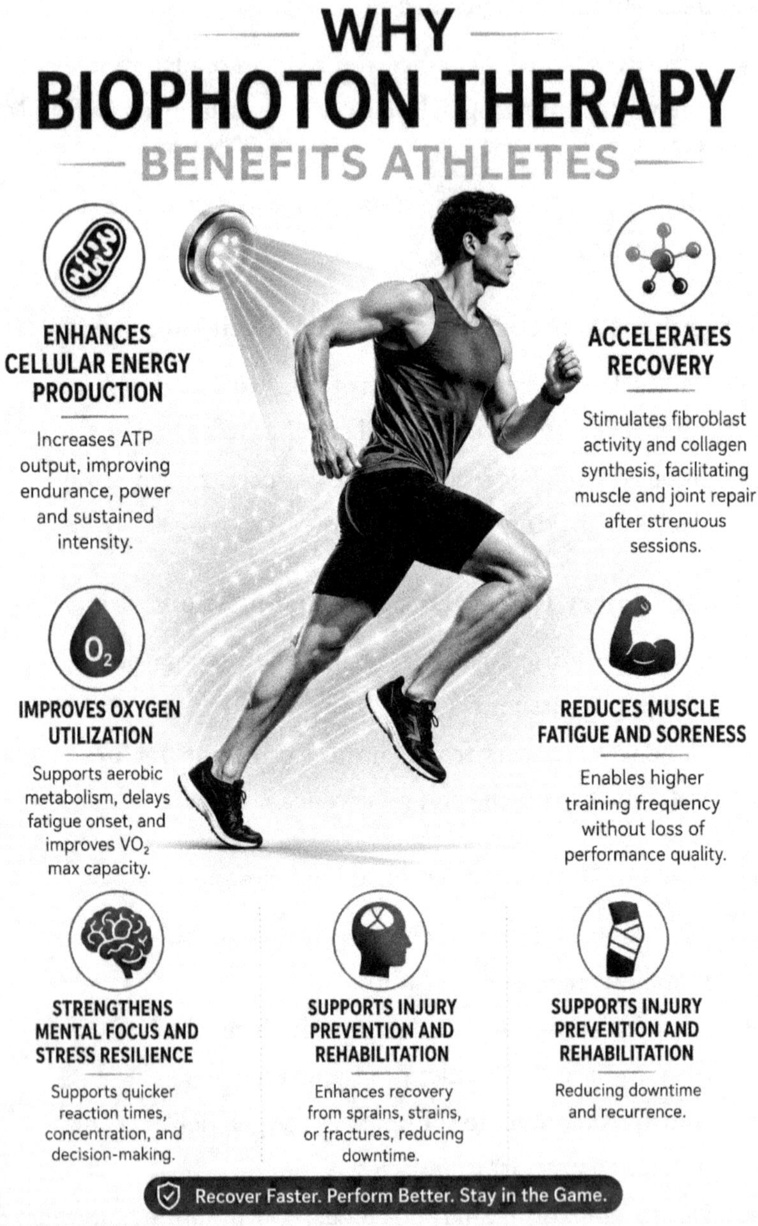

Figure 31.1. Why Biophoton Therapy Benefits Athletes. *Key mechanisms include enhanced cellular energy production, accelerated recovery, improved oxygen utilization, reduced muscle fatigue and soreness, strengthened mental focus and stress resilience, and support for injury prevention and rehabilitation.*

Potential Impact on Sports Performance

- Endurance Gains: Sustained peak intensity during training and competition.
- Strength and Power: Increased neuromuscular efficiency and muscular output.
- Faster Reaction Times: Optimized neural signaling improves reflex performance.
- Reduced Injury Rates: Faster recovery and stronger tissue resilience prevent career interruptions.
- Consistency Across Seasons: Enhanced recovery enables athletes to maintain their peak condition long term.

Case Studies and Observations

- Professional Athletes: Report greater stamina, shorter recovery times, and improved competition-day performance when using biophoton devices.
- Sports Teams: Integration into rehabilitation protocols has reduced injury recurrence and accelerated return-to-play.
- Observational Reports: Athletes describe enhanced focus, confidence, and stress resilience during high-stakes competition.

Integration into Athletic Training Programs

- Pre-Competition: Use of biophoton therapy to boost energy and sharpen mental readiness.
- Post-Workout Recovery: Reduces inflammation and accelerates repair cycles.
- Injury Rehabilitation: Complements physiotherapy by enhancing healing speed and tissue quality.

- Daily Training: Maintains resilience and energy balance during heavy training blocks.

Policy Recommendations for Sports Organizations

- Sports Medicine Adoption: Integrate biophoton therapy in elite training and rehabilitation facilities.
- Research Expansion: Fund clinical trials to assess effects on endurance, strength, and injury prevention.
- Education Programs: Train athletes, coaches, and therapists on safe use and protocols.
- Ethical Considerations: Ensure compliance with fair play standards and avoid misuse as performance "doping."

Conclusion

Biophoton therapy is emerging as a transformative innovation in sports performance science. By restoring mitochondrial efficiency, accelerating recovery, and enhancing mental resilience, it offers athletes a safe, drug-free tool for improving competitiveness. Its ability to reduce fatigue, improve endurance, and stabilize performance across entire seasons positions biophoton technology as a cornerstone of next-generation sports medicine.

References

1. Karu T. Mitochondrial signaling activated by red and near-IR radiation. *Photochem Photobiol.* 2008;84(5):1091–1099.

2. Hamblin MR. Mechanisms and applications of the anti-inflammatory effects of photobiomodulation. *AIMS Biophys* 2017;4(3):337–361.

3. Bjordal JM, et al. A systematic review of low-level laser therapy with location-specific doses for pain, inflammation, and tissue repair. *BMC Musculoskelet Disord.* 2003;4:1.

4. Chung H, et al. The nuts and bolts of low-level laser (light) therapy. *Ann Biomed Eng.* 2012;40(2):516–533.

5. Douris P. et al. Effect of phototherapy on delayed onset muscle soreness. *Photomedicine and Laser Surgery* 2006, 24(3):377–82.

6. Salehpour F, Cassano P. Transcranial photobiomodulation therapy for cognition and mood. *Neurophotonics.* 2021;8(2):022001.

CHAPTER 32

Biophoton Energy Enhances Horse Racing Performance

Elevating Speed, Strength, and Recovery Through Energetic Optimization

---

When internal light flows in harmony, movement becomes power. —**James Z. Liu, MD, PhD**

Introduction

Horse racing places extraordinary physiological and psychological demands on thoroughbred horses, requiring maximal strength, endurance, cardiovascular efficiency, and rapid recovery capacity. Traditional interventions—such as specialized diets, conditioning programs, and veterinary care—are essential but often insufficient to fully prevent fatigue, accelerate recovery, or reduce injury risks.

Biophoton energy therapy, a non-invasive and drug-free modality, offers a novel approach to enhance equine sports performance. By optimizing mitochondrial function, improving oxygen utilization, modulating inflammation, and supporting mental calmness, biophoton therapy may represent a paradigm shift in equine performance science [1,2].

Demands for Horse Racing

- Physical Strain: High-speed galloping produces muscle microtrauma, oxidative stress, and heavy joint loading.

- Injury Risk: Tendon strains, ligament damage, and stress fractures are frequent causes of downtime and career decline.
- Recovery Challenges: Elite horses must recover within short intervals to sustain consistent racing schedules.
- Mental Focus: Horses must remain calm and responsive to jockey cues in high-stimulation race environments.

Why Biophoton Energy Benefits Equine Performance

1. Boosting Cellular Energy Production

- Biophotons stimulate mitochondrial cytochrome c oxidase, enhancing ATP synthesis [1,2].
- Higher ATP output increases muscular endurance, sprint power, and sustained racing performance.

2. Accelerating Muscle Recovery

- Reduces exercise-induced cytokines (IL-6, TNF-α), mitigating inflammation [3].
- Promotes fibroblast activation and collagen synthesis, supporting faster tissue repair.

3. Enhancing Oxygen Utilization

- Improves microcirculation and capillary oxygen delivery.
- Increases aerobic capacity, delays fatigue onset, and supports prolonged speed maintenance [4].

4. Reducing Injury Risk

- Stimulates connective tissue remodeling and collagen production.
- Strengthens tendons and ligaments, reducing the risk of musculoskeletal breakdown.

5. Optimizing Mental Focus and Stress Resilience

- Influences neurotransmitter balance, lowering stress and anxiety.
- Promotes mental calmness, improving responsiveness to jockey guidance.

6. Strengthening Immune Function

- Enhances systemic resilience, lowering infection risk during intense training and racing cycles.
- Supports continuous training schedules and race readiness.

Applications for Horse Racing

- Pre-Race Preparation: Boosts ATP and primes horses for peak physical output.
- Post-Race Recovery: Reduces muscle soreness and accelerates tissue repair.
- Injury Rehabilitation: Speeds recovery from tendon, ligament, and joint injuries.
- Training Enhancement: Improves endurance, consistency, and performance across competitive seasons.

Scientific Insights into Biophoton Effects on Equine Athletes

- Improved Muscle Metabolism: Biophoton-treated muscles demonstrate enhanced glycogen storage and efficient energy turnover [4].
- Enhanced Lactate Clearance: Faster lactic acid removal reduces fatigue and soreness.
- Stronger Connective Tissue Integrity: Stimulates fibroblast activity, reinforcing tendons and ligaments.

- Better Cardiovascular Recovery: Enhances circulatory dynamics and accelerates heart rate recovery after exertion.

Case Studies and Observations

- Trainers report improved race times, greater stamina, and lower injury incidence in horses undergoing biophoton therapy.
- Horses show increased calmness and responsiveness in competitive environments.
- Rehabilitation periods for tendon and ligament injuries are shortened, reducing training disruptions and financial losses.

Integration into Equine Management

- Routine Conditioning: Biophoton sessions are included in regular training regimens.
- Veterinary Support: Used as adjunctive therapy for injury prevention and rehabilitation.
- Performance Monitoring: Coupled with biometric tracking for individualized optimization.
- Portable Devices: Mobile units allow stable- or racetrack-based pre- and post-race applications.

Future Research and Innovations

1. Optimizing Protocols: Identifying ideal wavelengths, dosages, and treatment schedules for equine physiology.
2. Performance Studies: Long-term trials across racing seasons to quantify outcomes.
3. Integration with Analytics: Combining biophoton data with veterinary diagnostics, gait analysis, and sports tracking.

Ethical Considerations

- Drug-Free and Non-Invasive: Aligns with equine welfare standards and anti-doping regulations.
- Fair Competition: Biophoton therapy is free of prohibited substances.
- Animal-Centered Care: Supports natural physiology without harmful interventions.

Conclusion

Biophoton energy therapy represents a transformative advance in equine performance medicine. By enhancing mitochondrial energy metabolism, accelerating recovery, strengthening connective tissues, and supporting mental resilience, biophoton devices provide thoroughbred horses with a safe, effective, and ethical method to achieve peak performance.

Its integration into equine training and veterinary care could elevate global standards in horse racing, promoting both competitiveness and welfare.

References

1. Karu T. Mitochondrial signaling activated by red and near-IR radiation. *Photochem Photobiol.* 2008;84(5):1091–1099.

2. Hamblin MR. Mechanisms and applications of the anti-inflammatory effects of photobiomodulation. AIMS Biophys. 2017;4(3):337–361. doi:10.3934/biophy.2017.3.337. Epub 2017 May 19.

3. Bjordal JM, et al. A systematic review of low-level laser therapy for pain, inflammation, and tissue repair. *BMC Musculoskelet Disord.* 2003;4:1.

4. Leal Junior EC, et al. Phototherapy on exercise performance and recovery: A systematic review. *Lasers Med Sci.* 2015;30(2):925–939.

CHAPTER 33

Biophoton Energy Increases Food Quality

Elevating Freshness, Vitality, and Nutrient Potential

When light moves in order through living systems,
nourishment becomes more complete.
—James Z. Liu, MD, PhD

Introduction

Maintaining the freshness, nutritional value, and safety of fruits and vegetables is a cornerstone of agriculture, food distribution, and global food security. Conventional preservation methods—refrigeration, controlled atmospheres, and chemical treatments—can delay spoilage but often carry limitations, including high energy use, added costs, and environmental impact.

Biophoton energy presents a sustainable, residue-free, and non-invasive approach to enhancing food quality. By stimulating plant cellular vitality, reducing oxidative stress, and extending shelf life, biophoton therapy has the potential to improve food systems from farm to consumer [1–5].

Importance of Freshness in Produce

- Nutritional Value: Fresh produce retains higher levels of vitamins (C, E, folates), antioxidants, and enzymes critical for human health [1].

- Consumer Appeal: Freshness dictates color, aroma, flavor, and texture—factors central to consumer purchasing decisions.
- Economic Impact: Post-harvest losses account for up to 30–40% of fresh produce globally, resulting in reduced farmer income and lower retail profits.
- Food Security: Shelf-life extension increases access to fresh produce, particularly in regions without advanced cold-storage infrastructure [3].

Why Biophoton Energy Preserves Food Quality

1. Enhances Cellular Vitality

- Biophotons stimulate mitochondrial respiration and chloroplast activity, sustaining metabolic processes and delaying senescence.

2. Reduces Oxidative Stress

- Lowers the activity of polyphenol oxidase and other enzymes that drive browning and degradation [2].
- Preserves chlorophyll, delaying yellowing and visible spoilage in leafy greens [1].

3. Improves Water Retention

- Supports aquaporin regulation, maintaining intracellular hydration.
- Reduces wilting and shriveling, preserving crispness in lettuce, cucumber, and leafy vegetables.

4. Activates Natural Defense Mechanisms

- Stimulates endogenous antioxidants such as superoxide dismutase (SOD) and catalase, enhancing resistance to microbial and fungal contamination [4].

5. Promotes Uniform Ripening

- Modulates ethylene signaling, improving ripening uniformity in climacteric fruits such as bananas and tomatoes.

6. Environmentally Sustainable

- Reduces reliance on chemical preservatives and refrigeration-heavy supply chains.
- Offers a low-carbon, low-waste alternative aligned with climate-resilient agriculture [5].

Applications Across Food Systems

- Post-Harvest Treatment: Application immediately after harvest slows degradation.
- Storage Facilities: Integrated systems in cold rooms and warehouses extend shelf life.
- Retail Environments: Grocery produce displays equipped with biophoton generators preserve consumer appeal.
- Households: Portable units maintain the freshness of fruits and vegetables in kitchens.

Scientific Insights into Biophoton Effects

- Chlorophyll Stability: Spinach and broccoli retain chlorophyll longer under photobiomodulation [1].
- Browning Inhibition: Apples and bananas treated with controlled light exposure show reduced enzymatic browning [2].
- Firmness Retention: Tomatoes and strawberries maintain greater firmness under LED and photobiomodulation treatments [3,4].

- Shelf-Life Extension: Studies show reduced microbial growth and longer freshness windows in fruits exposed to low-level light stimulation [4,5].

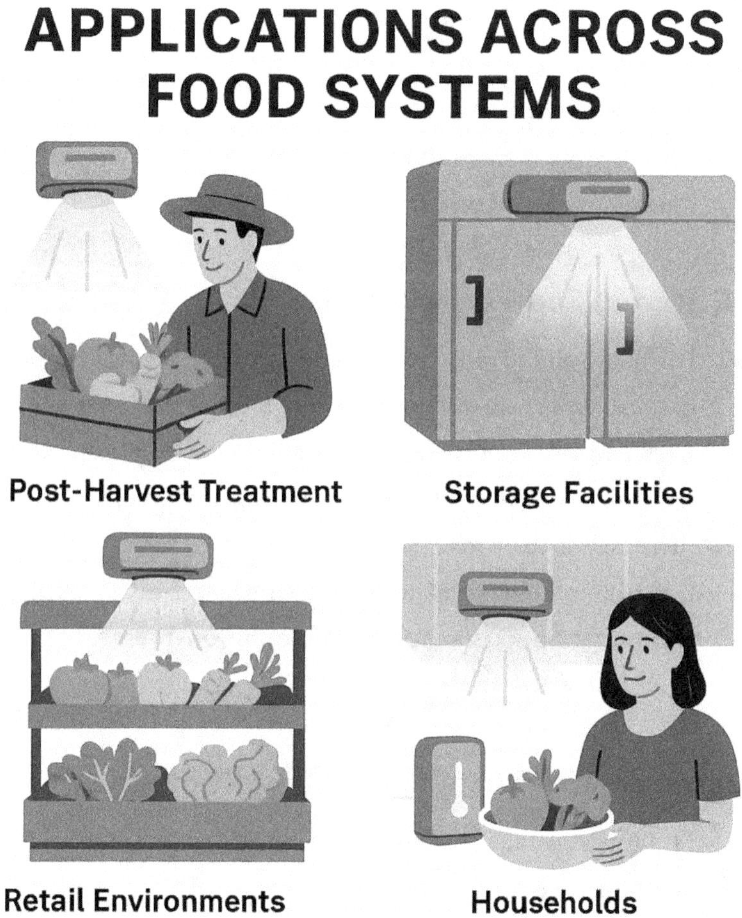

Figure 33.1. Applications Across Food Systems. *Infographic illustrating the applications of biophoton technology across various food systems, including post-harvest treatment, storage facilities, retail environments, and households, which each enhance the freshness and shelf life of fruits and vegetables.*

Potential Impact on Food Supply Chains

- Reduced Food Waste: Shelf-life extension directly lowers waste during distribution and retail.
- Energy Savings: Less reliance on high-energy refrigeration and atmosphere-controlled storage.
- Market Value: Fresher produce commands higher consumer trust and premium pricing.
- Food Security: Extends access to fresh food in regions with limited infrastructure.

Case Studies and Observations

- Farm-Level: Farmers applying biophoton technology post-harvest report slower spoilage and higher market quality.
- Retail-Level: Supermarkets using light-based preservation have observed improved longevity of leafy greens and increased fruit firmness.
- Consumer-Level: End-users describe better taste, texture, and nutrition satisfaction from biophoton-preserved produce.

Integration with Sustainable Food Practices

- Organic Agriculture: Offers a preservation method without synthetic chemicals.
- Supply Chain Efficiency: Extends transport windows, allowing longer-distance trade without sacrificing freshness.
- Eco-Friendly Design: Lower energy consumption reduces the environmental footprint compared to cold-chain heavy systems.

Conclusion

Biophoton energy therapy represents a paradigm shift in food preservation, offering a safe, eco-friendly, and highly effective way to maintain nutritional quality, freshness, and shelf life. By enhancing cellular vitality, reducing oxidative stress, and stimulating natural defense pathways, biophoton generators can complement or replace conventional storage methods.

Their integration into farms, storage facilities, retail systems, and homes may dramatically reduce food waste, cut energy use, and strengthen global food security, helping build a more sustainable and resilient food system for the future.

References

1. Yamauchi N, Watada AE. Chlorophyll and xanthophyll changes in broccoli florets stored under elevated CO_2 and/or reduced O_2 atmosphere. *Postharvest Biol Technol.* 1991;1(2):109–116.

2. Rocha AMCN, Morais AMMB. Polyphenoloxidase activity and total phenolic content as related to browning of minimally processed 'Jonagored' apple. *Int J Food Sci Technol.* 2001;36(2):121–127.

3. Wang Y. et al. Light-based improvement technology for postharvest fruits and vegetables flavor and regulation mechanism: a review. *Crit Rev Food Sci Nutr.* 2025;65(30):7010–7032.

4. Meng X, et al. Effects of light-emitting diode treatments on postharvest fruit quality and disease resistance in horticultural crops. *Food Qual Saf.* 2021;5(3):fyab023.

5. Hamblin MR. Mechanisms and applications of the anti-inflammatory effects of photobiomodulation. *AIMS Biophys.* 2017;4(3):337–361.

CHAPTER 34

Biophotons Increase the Yield of High-Value Agricultural Crops

Enhancing Photosynthetic Efficiency and Growth Dynamics for Greater Crop Productivity

---

Harnessing biophotons in agriculture transforms light into a precision growth technology—enhancing crop yield, nutrient density, and sustainability without compromising the planet's ecological balance.
—James Z. Liu, MD, PhD

Introduction

Agricultural productivity underpins both global food security and economic stability. Conventional yield-boosting strategies, including chemical fertilizers, pesticides, and genetic modification, have expanded food production, but at significant cost: soil degradation, biodiversity loss, and environmental pollution [1,7].

Biophoton energy, the ultra-weak photon emission associated with living systems [2], offers a clean, sustainable, and non-invasive approach to enhancing plant vitality. By stimulating photosynthesis, cellular metabolism, and stress-adaptive pathways, biophoton therapy has the potential to increase crop yields, improve nutritional quality, and reduce reliance on agrochemicals.

Agricultural Productivity Challenges

- Soil Degradation: Nutrient depletion and loss of organic matter reduce fertility in intensively farmed soils [1].
- Pests and Disease Pressure: Microbial and insect threats contribute to major crop losses globally.
- Climate Variability: Drought, salinity, and extreme weather increasingly destabilize yields [4].
- Resource Constraints: Rising demands for water and fertilizers highlight the need for more efficient growth systems.

Biophoton Mechanisms in Yield Enhancement

1. Enhancing Photosynthetic Efficiency

- Biophotons interact with chlorophyll molecules, improving quantum efficiency of photosystem II and overall photosynthetic rate [3,5].
- Result: Increased biomass accumulation and higher fruit/seed yield.

2. Improving Nutrient Uptake and Utilization

- Stimulates root elongation and branching, improving water and nutrient absorption efficiency.
- Supports higher productivity in limited-resource conditions.

3. Increasing Stress Resilience

- Biophoton stimulation upregulates heat-shock proteins, antioxidants, and osmoprotectants, enhancing tolerance to drought, salinity, and heat [4,6].
- Result: Yield stability even under climate variability.

4. **Balancing Plant Hormones**

- Modulates auxins, cytokinins, and gibberellins, optimizing flowering, fruit set, and grain filling.

5. **Reducing Dependency on Agrochemicals**

- Healthier, biophoton-energized plants show greater natural resistance to pathogens and insects, lowering pesticide needs.

6. **Accelerating Growth and Harvest Cycles**

- Biophoton stimulation shortens maturation cycles, enabling multiple harvests per season in high-value crops.

Applications for High-Value Crops

- Fruits: Larger size, richer color, and higher sugar content in grapes, citrus, and strawberries.
- Vegetables: Higher yields and nutrient density in tomatoes, cucumbers, and peppers.
- Grains: Increased productivity and stress resilience in rice, maize, and wheat.
- Medicinal Herbs: Enhanced secondary metabolites (polyphenols, alkaloids) in basil, ginseng, mint.
- Ornamentals: More vibrant flowers, improved resilience, and longer blooming periods.

Scientific Insights

- Chlorophyll Production: Biophoton energy promotes pigment biosynthesis, improving light capture and efficiency [5].
- Root Architecture: Plants exposed to coherent light develop deeper, more branched root systems, improving drought resilience.

- Stress-Resistant Genes: Light triggers expression of antioxidants and defense proteins, strengthening resilience [6].
- Increased Nutritional Value: Biophoton-enhanced crops show higher levels of vitamins, carotenoids, and polyphenols, improving human health outcomes [3,6].

The illustration below highlights the potential applications of biophoton-based agricultural enhancement in high-value crops. It demonstrates how ultraweak photon environments may support improved plant growth, nutrient density, resilience, and productivity across fruits, vegetables, grains, medicinal herbs, and flowering plants. The infographic emphasizes practical agricultural benefits such as enhanced crop quality, increased stress resistance, stronger immunity against common diseases, and improved yield potential. Together, these concepts present a vision of sustainable agriculture focused on healthier crops, higher economic value, and improved farming efficiency.

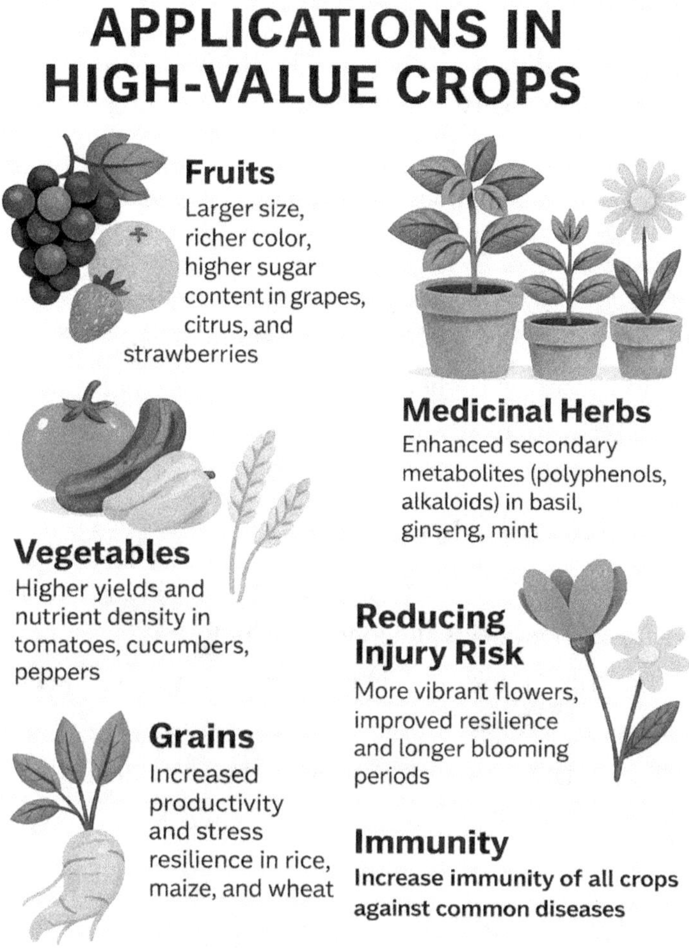

Figure 34.1. Applications in High-Value Crops. *Illustration summarizing the potential agricultural applications of biophoton energy across major crop categories. Reported outcomes include improvements in fruit size and sugar content, enhanced nutrient density in vegetables, increased productivity and stress resilience in grains, elevated secondary metabolite production in medicinal herbs, improved flowering performance, and strengthened crop resilience against common environmental stressors.*

Sustainable Agriculture Impact

- Higher Yields: Productivity gains without farmland expansion.
- Improved Quality: Better taste, nutrition, and post-harvest durability.
- Lower Inputs: Reduced demand for fertilizer and pesticides lowers production costs.
- Environmental Gains: Less chemical runoff, improved soil biodiversity, reduced carbon emissions [1,7].
- Food Security: Higher crop supply enhances affordability and availability globally [8,9].

Case Studies and Observations

- Greenhouse Crops: Biophoton-treated tomatoes and peppers show higher yields and longer shelf life.
- Orchards: Grapes and citrus fruits demonstrate enhanced sweetness, coloration, and uniform ripening.
- Field Trials: Farmers report reduced pest incidence and improved resilience in crops grown under biophoton exposure.

Integration into Agricultural Systems

- Seed Treatment: Pre-sowing biophoton exposure improves germination rates and seedling vigor.
- Growth-Phase Stimulation: Application during flowering and fruiting maximizes yield benefits.
- Post-Harvest Preservation: Extends shelf life and freshness during transport (see Chapter 28).
- Controlled Environments: Effective in greenhouses, hydroponics, and vertical farms, where biophoton fields can be precisely tuned.

Future Directions

- Optimizing wavelengths, intensity, and exposure protocols for crop-specific responses.
- Exploring synergies with regenerative and organic farming.
- Assessing effects on soil microbiome dynamics and plant–microbe communication.
- Developing portable biophoton units for scalable field deployment.

Conclusion

Biophoton energy represents a transformative, eco-friendly strategy for modern agriculture. By improving photosynthesis, nutrient use, and stress resilience, it offers measurable gains in yield, nutritional quality, and sustainability.

Integrating biophoton generators into mainstream farming could reduce environmental burdens, support food security, and elevate the economic value of high-value crops, positioning this technology as a cornerstone of resilient agriculture in the 21st century.

References

1. Foley JA, et al. Solutions for a cultivated planet. *Nature.* 2011;478(7369):337–342.

2. Popp FA. About the coherence of biophotons. *Macroscopic Quantum Coherence.* 1998;1(1):1–6.

3. Baker, N.R. Chlorophyll fluorescence: a probe of photosynthesis in vivo. *Annu. Rev. Plant Biol.* 2008;59:89–113.

4. Xu Y, et al. Plant adaptation to drought stress. *Plant Physiol.* 2010;154(1):125–131.

5. Lichtenthaler HK. Chlorophylls and carotenoids: pigments of photosynthetic biomembranes. *Methods Enzymol.* 1987;148:350–382.

6. Mittler R. Oxidative stress, antioxidants, and stress tolerance in plants. *Trends Plant Sci.* 2002;7(9):405–410.

7. El Bilali, H.; Strassner, C.; Ben Hassen, T. Sustainable agri-food systems: Environment, economy, society, and policy. *Sustainability.* 2021;13:6260.

CHAPTER 35

Biophotons Increase Fermentation for the Wine Industry

Enhancing Yeast Metabolic Efficiency and Fermentation Dynamics Through Light Coherence

---

When invisible light organizes living systems, refinement follows.

—James Z. Liu, MD, PhD

Introduction

Fermentation is the cornerstone of winemaking, determining not only the alcohol yield but also the sensory attributes—aroma, flavor, and mouthfeel—that define a wine's quality. This complex process relies on the metabolic activity of yeast (Saccharomyces cerevisiae) and, in later stages, lactic acid bacteria. Winemakers carefully control variables such as temperature, pH, nutrient availability, and oxygen exposure to optimize fermentation.

Despite advances in enology, persistent challenges remain, including:

- Sluggish or stuck fermentations caused by yeast stress.
- Inconsistent flavor development between batches.
- Yeast vitality loss under rising ethanol concentrations.

Biophoton energy, the emission and absorption of ultraweak photons by biological systems, offers a non-invasive, sustainable, and drug-free approach to address these challenges [1,2]. By stimulating yeast metabolism, enhancing fermentation efficiency, and stabilizing microbial ecosystems, biophoton generators present an innovative tool for the wine industry.

Fermentation in Winemaking

- Primary Fermentation: Yeast converts glucose and fructose into ethanol, CO_2, and heat.
- Secondary (Malolactic) Fermentation: *Oenococcus oeni* and other lactic acid bacteria convert malic acid into lactic acid, reducing acidity and enhancing flavor complexity.

Key variables influencing fermentation efficiency include:

- Temperature and pH.
- Yeast strain and nutrient balance.
- Stress factors such as ethanol buildup, oxygen limitation, or osmotic pressure.

Disruptions in these parameters often lead to reduced yield, uneven aroma development, or incomplete sugar conversion [3].

Why Biophoton Energy is Transformative

1. Stimulates Yeast Metabolism

- Biophoton exposure activates mitochondrial cytochrome c oxidase in yeast, enhancing ATP generation and overall metabolic activity [4,5].
- This shortens lag phases and accelerates sugar-to-ethanol conversion.

2. Improves Fermentation Efficiency

- Fermentation time is reduced without compromising ethanol yield.

- Promotes uniform fermentation kinetics across batches, increasing consistency.

3. Enhances Flavor and Aroma Profiles

- Biophoton energy modulates secondary metabolite pathways, enhancing the synthesis of esters, terpenes, and phenolics [6].
- Wines display richer bouquets, smoother palate structures, and balanced complexity.

4. Reduces Yeast Stress

- Increases tolerance to ethanol accumulation and temperature fluctuations.
- Maintains yeast vitality, minimizing risks of sluggish or stuck fermentation.

5. Increases Ethanol Yield

- Improves efficiency of sugar-to-ethanol conversion, maximizing alcohol production from the same grape must.

6. Promotes Microbial Balance

- Supports beneficial yeast and lactic acid bacteria populations.
- Helps suppress spoilage organisms, reducing reliance on sulfites and chemical additives [7].

Applications in the Wine Industry

- Red and White Wines: Improved fermentation speed and varietal expression.
- Sparkling Wines: Supports reliable secondary fermentation and carbonation stability.
- Organic/Natural Wines: Enhances native yeast performance, minimizing chemical interventions.

- Yeast Propagation: Increases starter culture vitality and robustness for predictable fermentation outcomes.

Scientific Insights

- CO_2 Output: Biophoton-treated fermentations show higher CO_2 release, indicating enhanced yeast metabolism.
- Yeast Viability: Maintains cell membrane integrity and extends survival under ethanol stress [4].
- Aromatic Compounds: Elevated production of fruity esters and floral terpenes enhances sensory qualities [6].
- Fermentation Rates: Studies on yeast photobiomodulation demonstrate faster kinetics without compromising quality [5,7].

Case Studies and Industry Observations

- Wineries implementing biophoton generators in fermentation tanks have reported:
    - Shorter fermentation times with equal or higher ethanol yields.
    - Improved sensory quality, richer aroma, smoother tannin integration, and greater varietal expression.
    - Reduced stuck fermentation, leading to fewer losses in premium wine production.

Integration into Winemaking Practice

- Fermentation Tanks: In-tank biophoton generators to support yeast metabolism during primary fermentation.
- Yeast Cultivation: Pre-treatment of inoculum cultures to increase yeast vigor before inoculation.

- Barrel Aging: Stabilizes microbial activity during malolactic fermentation and maturation.
- Bottling Stability: Reduces risk of undesirable post-bottling fermentations.

Future Directions

- Wavelength Optimization: Identifying the most effective bands (600–950 nm) for different yeast strains and grape varietals [5].
- Wine Aging Studies: Evaluating biophoton effects on polyphenol polymerization and flavor development during bottle maturation.
- Sustainability Benefits: Reducing refrigeration, chemical preservatives, and fermentation interventions.
- Collaborative Trials: Partnerships between wineries, biophysics laboratories, and enology research institutes will accelerate practical adoption.

Ethical and Industry Considerations

- Authenticity: No artificial additives are introduced—biophoton therapy preserves the natural heritage of wine.
- Sustainability: Aligns with eco-conscious, organic, and biodynamic winemaking practices.
- Compliance: Compatible with international wine standards and consumer transparency expectations.

Conclusion

Biophoton energy represents a paradigm shift in enology, combining tradition with modern biophysics. By stimulating yeast metabolism, reducing fermentation time, enhancing aroma profiles, and ensuring microbial stability, biophoton generators provide winemakers with a safe and sustainable tool to improve quality and competitiveness.

This innovation could redefine fermentation science in the wine industry, offering ecological benefits while elevating sensory excellence.

References

1. Popp FA. About the coherence of biophotons. *Macroscopic Quantum Coherence.* 1998;1(1):1–6.

2. van Wijk R, van Wijk EPA. An introduction to human biophoton emission. *Indian J Exp Biol.* 2005;43:445–457.

3. Fleet GH. Yeasts in winemaking. In: *Wine microbiology and biotechnology.* Harwood Academic Publishers; 1993.

4. Karu T. Mitochondrial signaling in mammalian cells activated by red and near-IR radiation. *Photochem Photobiol.* 2008;84(5):1091–1099.

5. Ann Liebert A. et al. Photophysical mechanisms of photobiomodulation therapy as precision medicine. *Biomedicines.* 2023 Jan 17;11(2):237.

6. Mendes-Ferreira A, Mendes-Faia A, Leão C. Growth and fermentation patterns of Saccharomyces cerevisiae under different nitrogen regimes and winemaking conditions. *J Appl Microbiol.* 2004;97(3):540–549.

7. Calabrò A, et al. Photobiomodulation as an eco-friendly tool to control microbial growth in food systems. *Innov Food Sci Emerg Technol.* 2020;65:102457.

8. Liu JZ, Gu HY, and Liu DR. Biophoton generators enhance germination, preserve produce and boost fermentation: A new frontier in quantum nutrition and agriculture. *Nov Tech Nutri Food Sci.* 2025;8(4). NTNF. 000691. doi: 10.31031/NTNF.2025.08.000691.

9. Liu JZ. Keynote presentation. Biophoton generators enhance global food yields: A new frontier in human nutrition and agriculture. *Marine-Future 2025 Aquaculture and Marine Ecosystem Sustainability*, September 22-23, 2025, Singapore.

CHAPTER 36

Biophotons Increase Fermentation for the Pharmaceutical Industry

Enhancing Yield, Stability, and Consistency in Fermentation-Based Drug Production

---

When energy within the cell is ordered, transformation becomes reliable.

—James Z. Liu, MD, PhD

Introduction

Fermentation remains a cornerstone of pharmaceutical manufacturing, supporting the production of antibiotics, vaccines, hormones, monoclonal antibodies, enzymes, and recombinant proteins. The efficiency, consistency, and scalability of fermentation processes directly influence drug availability, cost-effectiveness, and patient outcomes.

Conventional fermentation systems, whether microbial, mammalian, or hybrid bioreactors, face recurring challenges, including:

- Batch-to-batch variability in yield and potency.
- Culture stress due to pH shifts, ethanol buildup, or nutrient depletion.
- High contamination risk from competing organisms.
- Resource intensity, requiring energy-heavy sterilization and prolonged fermentation cycles [1].

Biophoton energy—ultraweak photon emission and absorption by living systems—offers a non-invasive, drug-free method to optimize fermentation. By stimulating cellular metabolism, stabilizing growth environments, and enhancing biosynthetic efficiency, biophoton generators can transform biopharmaceutical production into a more consistent, scalable, and sustainable process [2,3].

Fermentation in Pharmaceutical Production

Types of Pharmaceutical Fermentation

- Microbial fermentation: Used to produce antibiotics (e.g., penicillin, streptomycin), vitamins, and enzymes.
- Cell culture fermentation: Mammalian or insect cells cultivated to produce vaccines, monoclonal antibodies, and recombinant proteins.
- Bioreactor-based fermentation: Large-scale closed systems for optimizing sterility, growth conditions, and metabolic output [4].

Challenges in Conventional Systems

- Variable yields and potency across batches.
- Sensitivity to environmental fluctuations (temperature, oxygen, pH).
- Vulnerability to contamination by foreign microbes.
- Significant energy consumption for culture maintenance and sterilization [5].

Why A Biophoton Generator Is Transformative

1. Stimulates Microbial and Cellular Metabolism

- Biophoton exposure enhances mitochondrial cytochrome c oxidase activity and electron transport chain efficiency, accelerating ATP synthesis [6].

- Promotes faster cell division, higher biomass accumulation, and more efficient metabolite production.

2. Improves Fermentation Efficiency

- Reduces fermentation cycle times while maintaining drug quality.
- Enhances the productivity of antibiotics, enzymes, and biologics [7].

3. Enhances Product Consistency

- Promotes uniform metabolic conditions across culture volumes.
- Reduces variability in biologic potency, aiding regulatory compliance with GMP standards [8].

4. Reduces Stress on Cultures

- Stabilizes cellular performance under alcohol accumulation, nutrient shifts, or hypoxia.
- Increases cell viability and reduces apoptosis during extended runs [9].

5. Increases the Yield of Biopharmaceuticals

- Supports greater production of APIs, recombinant proteins, vaccines, and monoclonal antibodies.
- Scales yield upward without proportional increases in nutrient or energy input [10].

6. Supports Sustainable Manufacturing

- Decreases reliance on prolonged fermentation cycles, saving energy.
- Reduces the need for chemical stabilizers and additives [11].

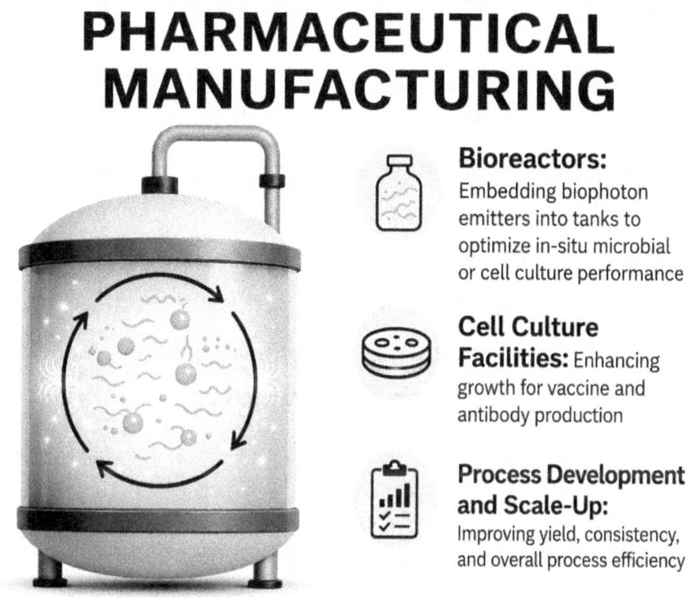

Figure 36.1. Infographic illustration of Biophoton Energy into Pharmaceutical Manufacturing. *Applications include bioreactors with embedded emitters, cell culture facilities for vaccine and antibody growth, process development during R&D scale-up, and quality control to stabilize fermentation and reduce variability.*

Applications in the Pharmaceutical Industry

- Antibiotics: Increased yields of penicillin, streptomycin, erythromycin, and next-generation antimicrobials.
- Vaccines: Higher cell culture density and antigen expression, enabling rapid scale-up in pandemic scenarios.
- Monoclonal Antibodies and Biologics: Improved titers, glycosylation fidelity, and stability in mammalian cell lines.
- Enzyme Production: Enhanced yield and enzymatic activity for biocatalysts used in drug synthesis.
- Probiotics and Nutraceuticals: Stronger survival, growth, and potency of pharmaceutical-grade strains [12].

Scientific Insights into Biophoton Effects

- Increased Biomass: Higher cell density and culture viability across microbial and mammalian systems [6,10].
- Enhanced Metabolism: Upregulated enzymatic activity and metabolite biosynthesis pathways.
- Improved Yield: Greater concentrations of recombinant proteins, secondary metabolites, and vaccine antigens [11].
- Reduced Contamination Risk: Favorable microbial balance discourages colonization by unwanted organisms [13].

Case Studies and Observations

Pharmaceutical companies adopting biophoton generators in bioreactors report:

- Faster production cycles with reduced batch times.
- Higher yields of antibiotics and therapeutic proteins.
- Reduced batch rejections due to improved consistency.
- Lower operating costs via reduced energy consumption.

These outcomes suggest a strong potential for biophoton therapy to reshape industrial fermentation economics.

Integration into Pharmaceutical Manufacturing

- Bioreactors: Embedding biophoton emitters into tanks to optimize in-situ microbial or cell culture performance.
- Cell Culture Facilities: Enhancing growth for vaccine and antibody production.
- Process Development: Incorporating biophoton modulation during R&D scale-up phases.
- Quality Control: Stabilizing fermentation conditions to reduce lot-to-lot variability.

Future Research and Innovations

- Parameter Optimization: Identifying ideal spectra (600–950 nm), intensities, and exposure protocols for different organisms [6,11].
- Regulatory Pathways: Integrating biophoton systems with FDA/EMA Good Manufacturing Practices (GMP).
- Precision Medicine Synergy: Supporting rapid, small-batch biologics for personalized therapies.
- Sustainability: Aligning with global "green pharma" initiatives to reduce carbon emissions and chemical waste [14].

Ethical and Regulatory Considerations

- Safety and Efficacy: All biophoton-optimized products must undergo rigorous testing.
- Regulatory Compliance: Full alignment with international pharmaceutical guidelines.
- Transparency: Reporting biophoton-related process modifications to regulators and stakeholders.

Conclusion

Biophoton energy represents a transformative advancement in pharmaceutical biotechnology. By stimulating cellular metabolism, reducing variability, and increasing yields, biophoton generators allow for faster, more consistent, and more sustainable production of life-saving medicines. As adoption expands, this technology could reshape global pharmaceutical supply chains, improving access to high-quality drugs while reducing environmental impact.

References

1. Crueger W, Crueger A. Biotechnology: A textbook of industrial microbiology. Sinauer Associates; 2000.

2. Popp FA. About the coherence of biophotons. Macroscopic Quantum Coherence. 1998;1(1):1–6.

3. van Wijk R. Biophotons and biocommunication. J Sci Explor. 2014;28(1):43–62.

4. Stanbury PF, Whitaker A, Hall SJ. Principles of fermentation technology. Elsevier; 2016.

5. Demain AL, Adrio JL. Contributions of microorganisms. Molecular Biotechnology. 01 Jan 2008;38(1):41–55.

6. Karu TI. Mitochondrial signaling in mammalian cells activated by red and near-IR radiation. Photochem Photobiol. 2008;84(5):1091–1099.

7. Hamblin MR. Mechanisms and applications of the anti-inflammatory effects of photobiomodulation. AIMS Biophys 2017;4(3):337-361. doi:10.3934/biophy.2017.3.337. Epub 2017 May 19.

8. Walsh G. Biopharmaceutical benchmarks. Nat Biotechnol. 2018;36:1136–1145.

9. Cassano P, et al. Transcranial photobiomodulation therapy in the cognitive rehabilitation of patients with cranioencephalic trauma. Photobiomodul Photomed Laser Surg. 2019 Oct 23;37(10):657–666.

10. Hakimiha N, Jahani Sherafat S, Laakso E-L and Fekrazad R. Photobiomodulation and the oral-gut microbiome axis: therapeutic potential and challenges. Front. Med. 2025;12:1555704

11. Chung H, et al. The nuts and bolts of low-level light therapy. Ann Biomed Eng. 2012;40(2):516–533.

12. Marco ML, et al. Health benefits of fermented foods: microbiota and beyond. Curr Opin Biotechnol. 2017;44:94–102.

13. Ailioaie LM and Litscher G. Probiotics, photobiomodulation, and disease management: Controversies and challenges. Int J Mol Sci. 2021 May 6;22(9):4942.

14. Ötvös SB et al. Advancing safe and sustainable by design practices in pharmaceutical manufacturing: The PHARMECO project. ChemSusChem. 2025;18(22):e202501218.

CHAPTER 37

You Are Light—Feed the Light

Embracing a New Relationship with Food, Energy, and Self

You are not just made of atoms; you are shaped by photons, guided by frequency, and sustained by resonance. Nourish yourself accordingly.
—James Z. Liu, MD, PhD

Light Is Life

Throughout this book, we have explored the science and soul of quantum nutrition. From mitochondrial photoreception to meridian signaling, from the coherent emissions of raw greens to the regenerative role of red light, biophotonics demonstrates that light is not merely a metaphor for life—it is life itself.

At the deepest level, you are not a machine destined to wear down. You are a field of vibrational intelligence, encoded in photons, communicating through frequency, and designed for coherence and renewal [1–3].

The central question of health is no longer 'What should I eat?' The real question is: *How can I align with the light I already am?*

A New Relationship with Food: Information, Not Just Fuel

Food is more than macronutrients; it is structured energy and information.

- Every bite carries encoded biophotonic signals that regulate cellular communication [1,4].
- Fresh plants retain the photonic memory of the sun, structured in chlorophyll and cellular water [5].
- Fermented foods pulse with coherent microbial light patterns that influence immunity and mood [6].

When you eat biophoton-rich food with awareness and gratitude, you do more than feed your body; you strengthen your biofield coherence.

A New Relationship with Energy: Coherence as the Source

True energy does not come from stimulants or supplements.
It arises from resonance and alignment.

You enhance your vitality when you:

- Receive morning sunlight to reset circadian rhythms and mitochondrial cycles [7].
- Drink structured water, which improves hydration and signal transmission [8].
- Sleep within coherent light fields that support melatonin release and tissue repair [9].
- Release emotional and environmental drains, restoring field symmetry.

Your body thrives when it is in frequency with its environment.

A New Relationship with Self: Remembering Wholeness

You are not broken—you are a coherent pattern of light sometimes obscured by noise.

Quantum nutrition is not about rigid control. It is about listening to your field.

The same frequencies that guide a sprouting seed also restore your organs. The same sunlight that grows food also grows you.

When you nourish yourself as light, research suggests you may:

- Improve repair and reduce oxidative damage [7,10]
- Support neuroplasticity and cognition [11]
- Enhance emotional balance and resilience [12]
- Slow or reverse biological aging through field coherence [13]

To live as a quantum being is to participate in a living circuit of light.

A Global Invitation: Feeding the Planet's Light

What happens when millions begin to eat, move, and live in ways that honor biophotonic nutrition?

- Hospitals evolve into centers of frequency-based care.
- Farms prioritize vitality and coherence over yield alone.
- Families cultivate environments of light, plants, pets, and shared presence.
- Nations transition from chronic disease management to planetary wellness.

Already, clinics integrating photobiomodulation, biophoton-rich diets, and coherence practices are reporting measurable benefits, from cardiovascular recovery to improved neurocognition [6–11].

Healing begins in each cell, but its resonance ripples outward—to families, communities, ecosystems, and the planet itself.

Remember This

- You are not only flesh, but you are also frequency.
- Your food is not only about matter, but it is a memory of sunlight and soil.
- Your daily choices restructure your biofield.
- Your light is not only for you, but it also uplifts the world.

Final Reflection

"The body is the lamp. The field is the flame. Light it with presence, and the whole being shines."

As you close this book, may you open a new chapter in your own life.

Feed yourself in a way that honors your light.
Move, rest, breathe, and eat as if you are already whole, because you are.

You are light.
Feed the light.
And illuminate the world.

References

1. Popp FA. About the coherence of biophotons. *Radiat Environ Biophys.* 1999;38(2):95–102. doi:10.1007/s004110050041.

2. Scholkmann F, Fels D, Cifra M. How ultraweak photon emission from living organisms is generated and used for intercellular communication. *J Photochem Photobiol B.* 2013;139:76–90. doi:10.1016/j.jphotobiol.2014.02.002.

3. van Wijk R. *Light in Shaping Life: Biophotons in Biology and Medicine.* 2nd ed. Meluna; 2014.

4. van Wijk EPA, van Wijk R, Bajpai RP. An analysis of spontaneous ultraweak photon emission of the human body. *PLoS One.* 2010;5(6):e11071. doi:10.1371/journal.pone.0011071.

5. Bohn T, Walczyk T, Leisibach S, Hurrell RF. Chlorophyll-bound phytochemicals and their bioavailability: implications for human nutrition. *Mol Nutr Food Res.* 2015;59(7):1237–1248. doi:10.1002/mnfr.201400734.

6. Buescher JM, Margaritis A. Microbial biophoton emission and fermentation dynamics. *J Photochem Photobiol B.* 2007;87(2):140–147. doi:10.1016/j.jphotobiol.2007.02.005.

7. Hamblin MR. Mechanisms and applications of photobiomodulation in health and disease. *AIMS Biophys.* 2017;4(3):337–361. doi:10.3934/biophy.2017.3.337.

8. Pollack GH. *The Fourth Phase of Water: Beyond Solid, Liquid, and Vapor.* Seattle, WA: Ebner and Sons Publishers; 2013.

9. Figueiro MG, Rea MS. Lack of short-wavelength light during the school day delays dim light melatonin onset (DLMO) in middle school students. *J Clin Endocrinol Metab.* 2010;95(5):2329–2334. doi:10.1210/jc.2009-2137.

10. Chung H, Dai T, Sharma SK, Huang YY, Carroll JD, Hamblin MR. The nuts and bolts of low-level laser (light) therapy. *Ann Biomed Eng.* 2012;40(2):516–533. doi:10.1007/s10439-011-0454-7.

11. Salehpour F, Mahmoudi J, Kamari F, Sadigh-Eteghad S, Rasta SH, Hamblin MR. Brain photobiomodulation therapy:

a narrative review. *Neurophotonics.* 2019;6(2):022003. doi:10.1117/1.NPh.6.2.022003.

12. McCraty R, Atkinson M, Tomasino D, Bradley RT. The coherent heart: heart–brain interactions, psychophysiological coherence, and the emergence of system-wide order. *Front Psychol.* 2019;10:1710. doi:10.3389/fpsyg.2019.01710.

13. Horvath S, Raj K. DNA methylation-based biomarkers and the epigenetic clock theory of ageing. *Nat Rev Genet.* 2018;19(6):371–384. doi:10.1038/s41576-018-0004-3.

Appendices

Glossary of Quantum Nutrition Terms

ATP (Adenosine Triphosphate). The primary energy currency of the cell is produced by mitochondria. ATP production is enhanced by biophoton input and red/near-infrared light.

Bioavailability. The degree to which a nutrient or substance is absorbed and made available to the body. In quantum nutrition, this also includes vibrational and photonic accessibility.

Biofield. An electromagnetic and quantum field surrounding and permeating the body, believed to regulate health and biological function. Also known as the human energy field.

Biophotons. Weak but coherent light emissions from biological systems, primarily from DNA in the nucleus and mitochondria. Biophotons are believed to regulate cellular communication and vitality.

Breath coherence. A state achieved when breathing patterns entrain heart rate variability and nervous system balance, leading to increased field order and emotional stability.

Circadian rhythm. The body's internal 24-hour clock is regulated by light exposure and biological cues. Synchronizing with natural light cycles is key to quantum nutrition.

Coherence. A state in which waves (light, sound, or energy) are in harmony and structured. Biological coherence reflects optimal health, communication, and order.

Deglycation. The removal or prevention of advanced glycation end-products (AGEs), which are harmful compounds formed when sugar binds to proteins. Light and fasting enhance deglycation.

Electromagnetic Field (EMF). Invisible fields of electric and magnetic energy. Excessive artificial EMFs can disrupt biological fields; grounding and biophotons can help restore balance.

Epigenetics. The study of how behaviors and the environment can influence gene expression without changing DNA. Light, food, and field exposure can have epigenetic effects.

Frequency. The rate at which energy vibrates. In quantum nutrition, all inputs (food, light, thought) are understood to carry specific frequencies that affect biology.

Grounding (Earthing). Direct skin contact with the Earth's surface, which transfers free electrons to the body and can reduce inflammation, stress, and EMF load.

Heart Rate Variability (HRV). A measure of the variation in time between heartbeats. High HRV indicates good coherence and autonomic balance.

Hydration (Structured Water). Water in a highly ordered form that stores and transmits energy. Found naturally in raw foods and formed near hydrophilic surfaces and in biophoton fields.

Light Nutrition. The concept that specific wavelengths of light (especially sunlight and red/NIR) serve as essential inputs for mitochondrial and systemic health.

Mitochondria. Organelles in cells are responsible for producing energy. Responsive to red/NIR light, oxygen, and raw nutrients.

Photobiomodulation (PBM). The use of low-level red or near-infrared light to stimulate healing, regeneration, and cellular function. Often used in biophoton therapy.

Photonic Food. Food high in biophoton emissions, typically raw, fresh, and organically grown. These foods carry the sun's coherence and vibrational intelligence.

Quantum Biology. An emerging field exploring how quantum principles such as tunneling, entanglement, and coherence apply to biological processes.

Quantum Nutrition. A systems-based approach to nourishment that includes not only biochemical content but also frequency, coherence, biofield alignment, and light.

Red Light Therapy. The therapeutic use of red (620–750 nm) and near-infrared (750–950 nm) light to boost mitochondrial energy, repair tissue, and reduce inflammation.

Resonance. The tendency of energy systems to vibrate in harmony. Healing often occurs when the body's frequency is brought into resonance with natural patterns.

Senescence (Cellular). A biological aging state in which cells cease dividing and emit inflammatory signals. Light and field therapies may reduce or reverse senescence.

Structured Eating. A meal rhythm that honors circadian and seasonal timing to optimize digestion, energy, and biophoton absorption.

Tesla BioHealer. A medical-grade device designed to emit concentrated biophoton fields to support the regeneration of the body's biofield and mitochondrial function.

Vibrational Healing. A therapeutic approach using frequency-based inputs (sound, light, breath, intention) to restore balance to the biofield and body.

Zero-Point Field. A quantum concept referring to the background energy field that permeates space. Thought to be the source of all energetic potential.

Food Biophoton Emission Index (Selected Examples)

Measuring the Light Stored in What We Eat

The more coherent light a food emits, the more it nourishes not only the body, but the field.
—James Z. Liu, MD, PhD

Biophoton emission from food is an emerging metric that reflects a food's **vitality, coherence, and informational richness**. This emission is not detectable by the naked eye but can be measured using photomultiplier devices and ultraweak photon emission (UPE) techniques.

Foods that are raw, organically grown, freshly harvested, and minimally processed generally emit **more biophotons**, making them **higher in quantum nutritional value**.

Below is a simplified index of selected foods based on documented biophoton emission studies (primarily referencing the work of Fritz-Albert Popp and others).

Food Item	Biophoton Emission Level	Notes
Raw sprouted mung beans	★★★★★	Among the highest; high metabolic activity, rich in enzymes and chlorophyll
Raw spinach (fresh-picked)	★★★★☆	High in structured water and photosynthetic pigments

Food Item	Biophoton Emission Level	Notes
Carrot (organic, raw)	★★★★☆	Strong emission due to β-carotene and fiber coherence
Apple (tree-ripened, organic)	★★★★☆	High emission when not stored long; carries strong plant information
Raw broccoli	★★★★☆	Contains sulforaphane and active enzymatic structures
Tomato (vine-ripened)	★★★☆☆	Emission decreases with storage; best when fresh and sun-ripened
Raw milk (grass-fed cow)	★★★☆☆	Higher than pasteurized; biophoton content affected by animal health
Fermented sauerkraut (raw)	★★★☆☆	Emits coherent photons due to live microbial activity
Cooked vegetables (lightly steamed)	★★☆☆☆	Emission drops due to heat, but some structure remains
Pasteurized juice (orange)	★☆☆☆☆	Low photon output due to processing and oxidation
Refined white sugar	☆☆☆☆☆	Virtually no emission; energetically inert
Processed snack foods (e.g., chips)	☆☆☆☆☆	No measurable emission; biophoton-depleted and pro-inflammatory

★★★★★ = Very High

★★★★☆ = High

★★★☆☆ = Moderate

★★☆☆☆ = Low

★☆☆☆☆ = Very Low

☆☆☆☆☆ = Negligible or None

Key Observations

- **Freshness matters**: Time from harvest directly affects photon emission.

- **Processing reduces light**: Pasteurization, frying, and refining strip food of its coherence.
- **Living foods emit light**: Sprouts, raw vegetables, and fermented foods are top sources.
- **Coherence reflects vitality**: The more structured a food's water and enzymes, the higher the emission.

Applications

Use the Biophoton Emission Index to:

- Select foods that enhance your energy field
- Design quantum-rich meal plans
- Educate others about the vitality of living nutrition
- Compare storage, cooking, and farming methods

Suggested Reading and Resources

Expand Your Knowledge of Light, Frequency, and Living Nutrition

Biophoton Science and Quantum Biology

1. Popp, Fritz-Albert – *Biophotonen: Das Licht in unseren Zellen (Biophotons: The Light in Our Cells)*
   A foundational text on the science of biophoton emission from living cells.
2. McFadden, John & Al-Khalili, Jim – *Life on the Edge: The Coming of Age of Quantum Biology*
   A compelling and accessible introduction to quantum effects in biological systems.
3. van Wijk, Roeland – *Light in Shaping Life: Biophotons in Biology and Medicine*
   A thorough exploration of how biophotons regulate biological function.
4. Pollack, Gerald H. – *The Fourth Phase of Water: Beyond Solid, Liquid, and Vapor*
   Breakthrough insights into structured water and its implications for energy and health.

Energy Medicine and Biofield Science

1. Rubik, Beverly – Articles on the biofield and energy-based healing
   Available via PubMed and *The Journal of Complementary and Alternative Medicine.*
2. Oschman, James L. – *Energy Medicine: The Scientific Basis*
   Explains the energetic mechanisms behind healing modalities like acupuncture, touch therapy, and light therapy.

3. Becker, Robert O. – *The Body Electric: Electromagnetism and the Foundation of Life*
   A classic exploration of the electrical nature of living organisms.

Consciousness and Coherence

1. Dispenza, Joe – *Becoming Supernatural: How Common People Are Doing the Uncommon*
   Merges neuroscience, energy medicine, and consciousness research.
2. Sheldrake, Rupert – *The Presence of the Past: Morphic Resonance and the Habits of Nature*
   Introduces the concept of energetic memory and field inheritance in living systems.

Light Therapy and Longevity

1. Hamblin, Michael R. (Editor) – Photobiomodulation in the Brain: Low-Level Laser (Light) Therapy in Neurology and Neuroscience
   Advanced insights on red/NIR light therapy applications.
2. David Sinclair, PhD – Lifespan: Why We Age—and Why We Don't Have To
   A cutting-edge look at genetic, metabolic, and field-level approaches to reversing aging.

Functional and Integrative Nutrition

1. Deanna Minich, PhD – Whole Detox: A 21-Day Personalized Program to Break Through Barriers in Every Area of Your Life
   Connects food, color, and energy centers in a holistic healing system.

2. Mark Hyman, MD – The UltraMind Solution and The Blood Sugar Solution
   A functional medicine approach to diet, detoxification, and brain health.

Tools and Technology

- Bio-Well® GDV Camera – Non-invasive biofield imaging device based on the work of Konstantin Korotkov.
- Tesla BioHealerTM – A biophoton-emitting medical device for field coherence and regeneration.
- Photobiomodulation Panels (Red/NIR Light) – Available from trusted brands like Joovv®, PlatinumLED, and Mito Red Light.

Journals and Databases

- *Journal of Photochemistry and Photobiology B: Biology*
- *Frontiers in Physiology – Biophysics and Computational Biology*
- *Journal of Biophotonics*
- *Alternative Therapies in Health and Medicine*

About the Author

James Z. Liu, MD, PhD

Dr. James Z. Liu is a pioneering physician-scientist at the intersection of quantum biology, regenerative medicine, and integrative nutrition. With dual doctorates in medicine and human nutrition, Dr. Liu brings a uniquely holistic perspective that bridges cellular science with energetic healing.

As the founder of several wellness innovation platforms, including initiatives in biophoton therapy and cellular communication, Dr. Liu has led groundbreaking clinical observations that demonstrate how light, structured water, and vibrational fields can support recovery from chronic illnesses, neurological conditions, and age-related decline—without invasive intervention.

His research and leadership have contributed to the advancement of biophoton devices, including FDA-registered tools used in clinics across the U.S. and internationally. He is also a recognized voice in the emerging field of quantum nutrition, which integrates light-based healing with whole-food science, consciousness medicine, and lifestyle alignment.

Beyond the lab and clinic, Dr. Liu is a passionate educator and advocate for a new healthcare paradigm—one rooted not in disease suppression, but in coherence, frequency, and the innate intelligence of the body.

When he's not writing or mentoring practitioners, Dr. Liu collaborates with forward-thinking technologists, farmers, and longevity researchers to help shape a future where food, light, and consciousness are understood as the primary medicines of life.

www.ingramcontent.com/pod-product-compliance
Lightning Source LLC
LaVergne TN
LVHW052043200926
848481LV00005B/1725